Who Says You Can't Change the World?

A Legacy of Love and Faith

By Barbara Davis

We, Tom and Paula Patterson, are happy to give Barbara Davis permission to write about our son, Andy, and his adventures in education in Mentor. We give her permission to use our correspondence, letters, items previously published in "The Up Side of Downs Newsletters," and pictures or other materials. We are honored that she wants to tell his story, and are so appreciative of the huge part she played in it.

Sincerely
(Signed) Tom and Paula Patterson

WHO SAYS YOU CAN'T CHANGE THE WORLD?
Published by Ambrosia Press

Copyright October 2005 by Barbara Davis
Cover art copyright October 2005 By Nick Meyer
Library of Congress Control Number: 2005934887

For information address: Ambrosia Press
ambrosia03@earthlink.net
2 Waban Road, Suite 3, Willowick, Ohio 44095

Hardcover ISBN 0-9729346-0-X
9780972934602

Paperback ISBN 0-9729346-1-8
9780972934619

SECOND EDITION

WHO SAYS YOU CAN'T CHANGE THE WORLD?

A Legacy of Love and Faith

Dedicated to Paula

An Exemplar of <u>LOVE</u>
For in the giving the best she had to make others better,
In that giving, became better herself.

And of <u>FAITH</u>
Along the journey from bearing a precious son with
Down syndrome to the fullness of his life . . . and others.

The reason for this work is twofold.   When the author asked Paula, "Aren't you pleased with Andy?"   Her face was one of pure rapture as she illumined the room with her, "Oh! Yes!" It is the light in that window of her face that tells people her heart is at home. Secondly, the work surfaced from the elementary principal's assurance to Andy's family that "we can teach him what he needs to know," coupled with her own growth and reflection of her feelings about him. She cared, she dared, and now, she must share!

Printed in the U.S.A.
by Vision Press Inc.
Painesville, Ohio

Contents

Chapter 1 - Coastal Sunrise
A New Son

"For the sailor without a destination, there *is* no favorable wind," declares the seasoned seafarer. This truth is written, framed, and posted front and center in the main passageway; not the passage to the captain's quarters, nor to the office of the CEO, but in the main hall of an American public school. A "favorable wind" will blow on the good school with the vision that **everyone** is teaching and **everyone** is learning in concert with one another.

The attractive and astute mother of Andy wholeheartedly believed the school's vision when she made her initial appointment with the somewhat new principal of the neighborhood elementary school. She explained that her three older children were graduates of this community school, and of course, she would like to enroll Andy in kindergarten next year. She knew that **everyone** was the operative word during this first conference.

She also knew that in 1954 Chief Justice Earl Warren *(Brown v. Board of Education)* had declared, "In these days, it is doubtful that any child may reasonably be expected to succeed in life if he is denied the opportunity of an education. Such an opportunity, where the state has undertaken to provide it, is a right that must be available to all on equal terms."

Andy's mother continued to explain a few more details about her son to the principal, sharing why her vision for him is imbedded with that of the school. "We were lucky because Andy was our fourth child, so we already knew how to be parents." They didn't need any of the self-help books found in vast arrays that occupy a great amount of space in today's bookstores and libraries.

Chapter 2 - Low Tide
Down Syndrome Diagnosis

"Andy was born on February 17, an unusually warm winter day." She continued, "During his first seven hours with us the joy of a newborn boy permeated the entire family. Then, just as fierce and wicked as the Ohio cold front sweeping in from the north, the sky tumbled down on all of us. We had to depend on medical experts, as Andy was taken away to a 'special' nursery. Was that the beginning of the reason I now hate the word 'special' when applied to Andy? I had lost the child I had just delivered to the medical profession. I went from being a practiced, calm, self-assured mom, to being panicked that I would not know what he would need, or how to give him what he had to have."

She continued, "After the diagnosis was made, that he had Down syndrome and congenital heart disease, I was told that there were wonderful people who would help develop his strengths, so the next step was to 'give' him to the interventionists! During Andy's first year I learned to rely on the 'experts' who designed his program and his activities, and his schedule of appointments."

Andy's parents knew almost right away when Andy was born, that something was different about his heart. The doctor's diagnosis was that he had an atria sepal defect (ASD). That meant that there was a hole between the upper two chambers of his heart. Since the oxygenated and non-oxygenated blood mix, it causes strain on the heart and lungs and must be fixed. Doctors did all sorts of tests; i.e., echoes, EEGs, and finally a catherization, because they do not always know everything before they operate to make repairs. They had said they would repair his heart when he was about two. But the tests proved he was sicker than they thought, and they decided to operate as soon as possible. Since his birthday was the next week, the family asked that the surgeons wait until after his birthday. He was admitted for surgery the day after he turned one. With this first operation his parents knew that the experts would see them through the surgery that would finally make him well! They assumed so much then - among other fantasies, they thought the experts would look at him in the same light that they did.

Andy's mother relates, "I was excited that he was going to be 'fixed' and he was finally going to be all ours! The day of the surgery was, of course, one of the longest of our lives. The surgeon was supposed to be one of the best, even though we didn't get to meet him before the operation. We will never forget the nurse taking him from us and carrying him down that hall and through the doors."

The next news was that his heart problem was more serious than had been diagnosed. The ASD became an "AV Canal." That meant that the mid-part of his heart, where the four chambers join, had holes so that the blood was all mixing. The valves of his heart were also formed differently than most, so he was patched, stitched and repaired as much as they could. After about four and one half hours, he was taken to the pediatric intensive care unit (PICU).

Andy's mother is a nurse so she was prepared for all the tubes and equipment attached to him when they first saw him. Dad was not, so it was extremely difficult for him. "But all I saw was the pink! His cheeks were actually pink, and it was then I realized how bad his color had always been. We could tell that he heard us, because when we talked, tears trickled down from his closed eyes," reiterated Andy's mother.

The hospital was very busy at this time. Beds were at a premium in the PICU, so as soon as patients showed improvement, they were evaluated to see if they could go to a regular floor. Andy's family was assured that he would be in the intensive care for at least 48 hours; he was transferred to a regular unit in less than 36 hours. The surgeon needed his bed for a case he was doing that day. As they left PICU, his nurse warned the family to really watch him, as he was not comfortable with the move.

Andy struggled mightily that day. Although he was awake, he was not moving except to breathe. His breathing was labored and noisy, and the pink was all gone. The surgeons did not visit him that day at all. The cardiologists did not come in until the late afternoon. They were not worried, saying that after all, these kids (with DS) have low tone. They did not know Andy, and did not know how active he usually was!

"We were up most of the night as I tried everything to make him more comfortable. By morning, I was very worried, and told everyone who would listen that I want a doctor to come in and see him STAT (medical for NOW)! Finally a student nurse brought in her preceptor (the teaching nurse) who listened to my concerns, and had the resident come right in. Although that resident didn't know us, he did acknowledge that moms are usually right about their kids, and ordered some tests. When we went for the EEG, the technician who knew Andy asked why he was breathing like he was, and when I dissolved into tears, she called the head cardiologist to come immediately.

"It turned out that Andy was in severe congestive heart failure. He had gained over five pounds in 24 hours, because the fluids were backing up in his body. His heart didn't have the strength to pump hard enough to move his blood through his kidneys. His heart ballooned to almost twice its size, and his liver was greatly enlarged. He was not conscious, and didn't even move when they drew blood. His dad remarked that he was getting used to having that done; I knew how very sick he was when there was no response to that."

The surgeon was called, and said that they had tried to see Andy the previous day, but hadn't been able to find where he had been moved. He was taken back to PICU, given mega drugs to help him, and finally was closely supervised as he should have been on the previous day. He began to improve towards evening, and after a few days, was really better enough to be sent to a regular room. The one-week stay kept being extended. He remained on oxygen, and continued to have ups and downs on the road to recovery. He spiked high fevers, and the dreaded pneumonia appeared also. He was not moving much, and could not sit up or hold his head up. The doctors said, "Well, he has Downs, doesn't he?" When Andy's mother explained that he usually could stand alone, they called for physical therapy and occupational therapy to help him regain his skills. Actually, he hadn't lost them; he was just too sick to do anything!

Finally the antibiotics took care of the pneumonia, and three heart medications got his heart working better. After almost three weeks, Andy came home! His mother says as they drove off, "I did love the nurses we had, and I was actually saddened that we would never need to come back, and would never see any of them again. I assumed he was cured!"

No! He wasn't!

Although after two years he was off his heart medications, his lungs had been permanently damaged. He contracted severe pneumonia several times over the next years, requiring hospitalization for treatment. He was also diagnosed with asthma, and was considered to have both obstructive and restrictive airway disease. His heart seemed to work well enough until he was in eighth grade. Another bout with pneumonia sent him to the hospital, and as he struggled to overcome that, his heart again went into failure. When it was back to PICU, the family realized he really wasn't fixed at all, but that this would be a continuing risk for him.

He had many other surgeries and hospitalizations as a young child. Although some were more involved than others, the family joked that they were rebuilding him, one section at a time! It wasn't a joke of course, but they knew that they had to get his health to his optimal state in order for him to get on with his life. They soon learned to expect the unexpected, and to prepare for slow healing times and complications. They confided, "We even learned to listen for the other shoe to drop when things were going too well!"

"In addition to the serious illness and surgeries, Andy's immune system doesn't work as well as most, so he had what seemed like endless ear infections, respiratory infections, and colds. Since illnesses triggered his asthma, winter was often a vicious cycle of doctor visits and antibiotics. Andy seemed to get things our other kids never had, like croup; he and

Megan shared numerous episodes of strep back and forth. The amazing thing was how he kept going. Even when he was sick, he would work on his sight words, counting, coloring, and learning new things. Since he had never known the usual good health we take for granted, it was simply standard ritual that he had to take medicine, see doctors, and go to the hospital. It was simply his way of life. He did have extreme fear of needles, blood draws, and doctors he did not know. Although it has lessened as he has grown, blood and needles are still major difficulties for him. He isn't just scared; he is terrified!"

His last medical diagnosis came when he was in first grade, when we saw a neurologist who thought he had Attention Deficit Disorder (ADD). A trial of Ritalin proved the doctor to be correct in his diagnosis, and Andy has taken this medication ever since. It was interesting that his first grade teacher wrote a note after the first week he was taking Ritalin. It seemed to her that "Andy had had a sudden spurt, and had really matured this week." She did not know he was taking it, so it was an unbiased opinion. On the few days he didn't take it, a note from the teacher asking if something was wrong as he had been so off the wall that day! The family has tried several different medications, and all have had some side effects, but the results certainly outweigh any of the side effects. Ritalin, or the other medications have enabled him to learn as much as he has learned, for without them he just cannot concentrate or focus on what he is doing. Since they also help control impulsive behavior, he is a much better citizen because of his medications.

"When he was so sick the staff blamed all his symptoms on his Down syndrome. They would not listen to me that he was very ill. Again and again during the course of the hospitalization when there was no one but me to stand up for him, to believe in him, to explain him . . . it was right then that I knew that deep inside I would find the strength and determination to see him through all that might be, and have the courage to make him my child again. Time and time again I have had to remind myself of that covenant, and that Dad and I are his parents who have promised to preserve and protect the person he is."

They kept their promise, and in so doing, it led them to the principal's office. Earlier that same week, serious risk-taking had been the topic of a staff development seminar at the neighborhood school. The new principal, in further expansion of her vision of a good school, encouraged adults and students to take risks, and to provide a safety net for those who do. "Adults must model risk-taking, and provide avenues for risks and for doing things differently," she explained.

Now right here, sitting before the principal, was risk-taking personified in Andy's mother. After her affirmative creed to "preserve and protect" the person called Andy, she was willing to hand him over to the school, where her maternal instincts told her he would survive and thrive! She continued by sharing fresh insight into her focused vision.

"My child will live in the real world after he is finished with school. He needs to know how to function in that real world. People in that real world will need to know him, and will need to know how to deal with the unique aspects of him. If he is to live in the real world that I envision for him, he must grow up in the real world of childhood, which I see in our community, as the neighborhood school. Going to school together, studying the same subjects in the same books as all his other classmates, getting ready for the same concert or play, planning for Open House, working on the same projects, etc., makes a child 'one of the gang' as nothing else can! This is my goal for Andy!"

Her goal had not been created through happenstance, she explained. "During these first five years of living with Andy, we learned that the dreams we had for him were not as impossible as we had thought. It seemed that the sadness of what might have been was our doing; we were setting limits, not thinking of how we could provide opportunities to accomplish what might be. The limitations had been created early on when we were told the details of his medical problems and of the need to find a program for his special needs. We heard lots of 'He probably won't,' 'it will take him a long time to,' and 'he might never.' We were overwhelmed with advice and opinions, and with grief, and with love for this little bundle of humanity. But Andy has proved strong and brave, and this toughness inspires us to be the same for him. Now we must make sure that Andy has the opportunity to try what he wants to do. This means knocking on doors, and forcing change on institutions and on people who don't always want to try something different. But without the opportunity to try, where would any of us be? Sure, we've mistakenly 'pushed' a lot of 'pull' doors, but I could conquer the world when he looks up at me with big brown eyes and says, 'We pals, Mom!'"

The author is reminded of Frank Ellis, who lost both his legs in World War II. In his book, <u>No Man Walks Alone</u>, Ellis writes, "Every single one of us is handicapped - physically, mentally, socially, and spiritually - to some degree; and although we seldom think about it, the person without faith has a far greater handicap than the person without feet" (Ellis, 1968).

Andy attended early intervention classes at a nearby county-run school for children with disabilities, the only early intervention available in 1984. He had a team of teachers, one of whom was excellent, but several who held a view of children with disabilities that fate had limited their potential, and keeping them in programs separated from the mainstream of life was the best solution to their "problems." This was difficult for Andy's parents, new to the "disability club," who believed that for Andy to live in the real world he must be educated in the real world!

They withdrew him after reviewing his "education plan" for the forthcoming year, when he would be two. He would ride the bus to classes every day, stay in school from 9 a.m. to 2 p.m. so he could watch "Sesame Street," have lunch, a nap, and ride the bus home again. Andy's mother stated, "This was not the life I had expected for our fourth child. I wanted to give him lunch, hold him on my lap to watch 'Sesame Street,' take him outside and play, and watch him learn the things I would teach him." So without a real plan, they left this school with new knowledge and a humble appreciation that Down syndrome was not the worst thing that could happen to a child. *They would not allow the death of their dream for Andy!*

One would have to believe that it was more than coincidental that their favorite teacher had taken a leave from the school to start her family about this same time. She decided not to return to the formal school program after her baby arrived, and accepted their invitation to tutor Andy on a private basis. She guided the family as they worked to keep him as close to the typical pace of development as they could, and acted as a sounding board as they considered all of Andy's needs. Karen continued working with Andy until he was almost four, but because of her husband's job transfer her family relocated to California. Andy's family was grateful to her, not only for her assurance that they were meeting his educational needs, but for her role as a guidance counselor as they traveled their new and unusual path.

Andy then attended a new program for toddlers at Hershey Montessori School. He attended the play group two mornings a week, while the mothers of all the children chatted in an adjoining room and watched all that was going on. Each week a teacher spoke to the mothers to explain what the direction the play would take, and how they could continue the experiences at home. This was a wonderful experience for Andy! He could do almost all the things his classmates could do, and the teachers helped him out with the things that were hard for him. He didn't speak as well as the other children, but they were great models for him, and his speech continued to develop.

About mid-year Andy's mother mentioned something to the other moms about his disability. She wanted them to know that it was fine to discuss it, which they had wanted to do. Without reserve they shared their feelings about having Andy with their child. Without exception, they were happy Andy was there. A few of them had known people with Down syndrome, and they had some inspiring tales to relate. One knew an adult with DS who could drive. Andy's mother began to believe more and more that if some children with DS could do certain things, there was nothing to make her think that Andy couldn't also do them. Andy missed three weeks of school in March of that year because he had surgery. During that time, all of the children sent cards and little gifts, and had a party for him when he returned to school.

Also in March, Andy's family had to decide what they would do for the next year. Teachers repeatedly told them that Andy needed socialization (sisters and brother don't count). They determined that he would start preschool at the ripe age of three. Although the Montessori program offered a three-year-old class, it was five mornings a week and the family felt that it would be too much for their three-year-old. The school personnel were willing to have Andy attend, and were sorry when he did not.

The teacher told Andy's mother not to underestimate his capabilities. She related, "He already knew what a bird was, and she told me that there was good reason to think that he would able to learn that some birds are cardinals, and some are robins, and others, blue jays. Andy's mother says, "I don't remember her name, but I remember her spirit, and it inspired me to continue on our path!"

The church preschool, where big sister Megan had attended, was Andy's next education experience, and it was right in his own back yard. His mother was uncertain whether or not they could enroll Andy. At a nursery school fair, as she was wandering around looking for a place that would take him, the director of the church preschool said if she wanted Andy to come there, he would be welcome. "Church members have preference," she added (as if she needed any encouragement other than them welcoming him)!

Andy attended preschool at the church for the next three years, at first two afternoons a week and then three afternoons. Andy did everything the other children did. Sometimes he did it with hand over hand assistance, sometimes alone, and sometimes he needed complete help. But he followed the rules, used the bathroom, had snacks, lined up, and participated in the Open Houses and other programs.

Each teacher worried that he would be unable to do what the next class required (a common thread throughout his entire education journey). Each year, however, Andy became more mature and capable, and was able to master most all that the other students did. Informal communication between home and school was essential before classes started and throughout the school year.

The daily contact with other children his age, many who have continued as friends today, probably helped him become who he is almost as much as all the work the teachers did. He wanted nothing more than to do whatever the others were doing, and he gave it his all to try. Because of the other children, he learned to line up, obey the teacher, share, play and follow the playground rules, hang up his coat, carry his book bag, say hello and goodbye to the teacher, and most of the skills he would need for his next school.

While he was in preschool, he always had a tutor to work on specific learning skills. After Karen relocated, upon the advice of the local school system, Andrea was with Andy until he went to elementary school. Andrea decided that teaching him sight words would be a good foundation for his learning to read. Andy's mother was thrilled that she thought he would be able to read, and believed that the sight words he learned were wonderful! He counted, learned shapes, colored, learned colors, and began reading with Andrea.

Because of Andy's low muscle tone, he was enrolled in a daily swimming program. The swimming instruction not only taught him an important life skill, but strengthened his muscles, increased his endurance, and strengthened his heart. His mother feels that the swimming saved his life after heart surgery. He had many complications after surgery, and had his heart not been strengthened, it would not have been strong enough to withstand all that had happened to him.

Additionally, he began taking speech at Cleveland State University; this continued for four years three times a week. He had excellent therapists there, and made much progress! He also had physical therapy and occupational therapy at Rainbow Babies and Children's Hospital in Cleveland during this time. Four days a week, he went to Cleveland for some sort of therapy, and then rushed back to Mentor for preschool in the afternoon. It was quite a schedule for a three-year-old! He and mom had a lot of "car time" together, and went singing through tape after tape of "Sesame Street" songs, and Sharon, Lois and Bram songs. All the singing helped with his speech development almost as much as the speech lessons. "By the time school started, we were having real conversations on those trips. Although I was happy to stop driving in all sorts of Northern Ohio weather, I was sad when those trips were over. My poor little baby with Down syndrome had grown into a most interesting and capable human being," Andy's mother boasted.

It is difficult for one to believe that prior to the passage of P.L. 94-142 (1975) children in Ohio were barred from a public education if, after submitting to an I.Q. test, they fell below a specified benchmark. In 1970 a mother of a retarded child was called to come and take her child out of school on the third day of her kindergarten experience. The principal at that time informed her that her daughter did not belong there! One wonders how often this had occurred.

This was the same school where Andy would attend exactly twenty years later. This was the same district, which these same two decades later, at the request of the Ohio Board of Education published its policy. "We, as an expression of our commitment to provide a free appropriate public education for children with disabilities in accordance with state and federal laws, rules and regulations, do hereby resolve to implement the following policies: It shall be the policy that the child with a disability and his/her parent shall be provided with safeguards, as required by law, throughout the identification, evaluation, and placement process, and the provision of a free appropriate public education to the child . . . It shall be the policy that the education of children with disabilities shall occur in the least restrictive environment (LRE); individual education programs (IEP) and services shall be appropriate and designed to meet the unique needs of each child with a disability; to the maximum extent appropriate, children with disabilities shall be educated with children who do not have disabilities; separate schooling, or other removal of children with disabilities from the regular educational environment, shall occur only when the nature or severity of the disability is such that education in regular classes with the use of supplementary aids and services cannot be achieved satisfactorily."

The IEP has become so commonplace (yet functional) that an anonymous writer has scribed:

IEPs According to Dr. Seuss

Do you like these IEPs?

I do not like these IEPs, I do not like them, Jeeze Louise,
We test, we check, we plan, we meet, but nothing ever seems complete.

Would you, could you like the form?

I do not like the form I see, not page 1, not 2, not 3,
Another change, a brand new box, I think we all have lost our rocks.

Could you all meet here or there?

We would not all meet here or there, we cannot all fit anywhere.
Not in a room, not in the hall, there seems to be no space at all.

Would you, could you meet again?

I cannot meet again next week; no lunch, no prep, please hear me speak.
No, not at dusk; no, not at dawn; at 4 p.m. I should be gone.

Could you hear while all speak out? Would you write the words they spout?
I could not hear, I would not write; this does not need to be a fight.

Sign here, date there, mark this, check that;

Beware the student's ad-vo-cat(e).

You do not like them, so you say;
Try again! Try again! And you may.

If you will let me be, I will try again, you will see.

Say!

I almost like these IEPs; I think I'll write 6003,
And I will practice day and night, until they say, "You got it
right!"

Andy's mother and the principal were well aware of the enactment of
"The Education for All Handicapped Children Act" *(P.L. 94-142).* It is of
interest, or what this principal called synchronicity, that "The Individuals
with Disabilities Education Act" (IDEA) was passed the year Andy
entered his neighborhood school, and its major amendments were enacted
the year he graduated from the school. The amendments, dedicated to
higher standards, coincided with much of the common sense the school
had been practicing; i.e., 1. Zero Rejection (all students will be educated);
2. Free Appropriate Public Education; 3. Related Services (busing,
occupational and speech therapists, tutors, counselors, etc.); 4. Least
Restrictive Environment (regular classrooms); 5. Identification and
Evaluation; and, 6. Procedural Safeguards. However, laws can take years
to be implemented for an individual state, district, school, or student.

Just recently (June 26, 2003) a Cleveland Plain Dealer headline read
"Pledge for Disabled Pupils Cut in Half." "Lawmakers who said they
would dramatically boost spending on education for children with
disabilities have cut back on their pledge, agreeing yesterday to provide
less that half the increase touted in April." Congress in 1975 set
requirements for educating children with disabilities, laying out expensive
mandates through what is now called IDEA. It promised to put up 40
percent of the cost, but never has provided near that amount. Schools
were hopeful this spring as Congress worked on renewing IDEA and

pledged a $2.2 billion increase for 2004. That was modified to a $1 billion boost, for a total appropriation of $9.9 billion. The article concludes, "The House will try to step up special education spending again. But you have to understand, we're under special circumstances this year. We've had a war that we've had to fund." The conclusion from the above sparks a satirical mockery in the mind of the author. Very often we see the following posted here and there in schools: "Someday they'll have to hold bake sales to build bombers."

In an excellent Phi Delta Kappan article, "No Child Left Behind: Costs and Benefits," William Mathis reviews the No Child Left Behind Act (NCLB), signed by President Bush in 2002. The promises exceeded reality, and there remained hard questions about costs and adequacy of resources. Mathis concludes, "States and districts must work with federal officials – elected and appointed – for the repeal or massive revision of the NCLB law so that it provides a workable accountability system. This system must include comprehensive and democratic conceptions of educational goals rather than a narrow reliance on tests. Finally, educators must embrace accountability. We must work to ensure that no school provides substandard, inadequate, or inequitable educational programs. We must do so not because it is politically expedient but because it is what we owe the children, our society, and ourselves" (Mathis 2003).

To retract "Tom and I did pretty much as we were told when Andy was first born. We went to Early Intervention, we started swimming classes, we made all the medical appointments, we listened to what people were telling us about Andy's life, and most of the time we believed them. But when I looked into Andy's eyes, there was a gleam that begged, 'Look at me! I can do anything I set my mind to! I am FINE!' I could not - and still cannot - reconcile those eyes with all the 'he will nevers' that we were being fed.

"When Andy was about 18 months old, we joined the National Down Syndrome Congress (NDSC), a national group for parents with children with Down syndrome. The NDSC was having a convention in Anaheim, California, that first year we joined. The bonus was the location -

Disneyland! I had dreamed of going there since I was about ten and now finally, because of Andy, I was going. This was the first of many things that we got to do, or places we got to see, or people we got to meet, because of Andy.

"Because most of my concerns were medical, I attended workshops that discussed the latest medical research as it applied to children with Downs. One researcher stated that with all the interest in DNA and gene mapping, he was sure that in about ten years, the chromosomes would be mapped, and they would know which genes would cause Down syndrome. I asked if it would help those who were already born, and he assured me it would. So, if we could just keep Andy going until he was about twelve, there could be a cure! His belief was a bit optimistic, for sure, but that idea kept me going during some really dark periods!

"Tom, however, went to whatever sounded interesting at the moment. He heard dads talking about their children having tongue reduction surgery to help with the speech difficulties many people with DS have. This also changed the 'tongue hanging out' appearance associated with the syndrome. Hummmm. . .were there more things we didn't know about that might help him?

"The next day Tom went to a seminar on rights. He talked excitedly on the way to San Diego during the next leg of our journey after the end of the conference. He spoke about a law that insured that children could get help in school, even if they couldn't see or hear, or sit up. This was so new to us that we didn't even know the name of the law, or how we might find out more about it.

"The next fall, I talked with the principal of our neighborhood school. He explained about the Individual Education Program (IEP) that would guarantee Andy could get what he needed educationally, and that he thought there was no reason he could not get his education at Center Street Village School. Wow! I had no idea that was a possibility! I had never known any children with disabilities at the school, but I listened well to this principal.

"Another November and another NDSC conference in Washington, D.C. featured the keynote speaker, Lou Brown, of the University of Wisconsin. His topic was inclusion, which meant that children with disabilities went to school where they would have gone, had they had no disability, and they shared classrooms, bus rides, and teachers with those who had no disabilities. **Everyone** was included in the neighborhood schools. If a student needed support to learn in that classroom, it was written in his IEP, and the service was delivered in the regular classroom.

"This was our awakening! The lights came on, and we realized this was what we wanted for Andy." Mr. Brown spoke of the importance of the neighborhood school as the starting point for real acceptance into society. He said that when kids grow up with all sorts of other kids, they know how to deal with each other. That continues into adulthood.

Much later, when Andy's Mother was a new parent contact for "The Up Side of Downs," she got a phone call from a dad who knew he was going to have a son with Down syndrome. His wife was about 20 weeks pregnant when they learned the facts of the baby's life. He was calling for advice. She reiterated, "Usually when parents call, they are trying to decide whether to keep the baby or not. I gingerly probed to learn if this was his reason for calling. I asked if he knew much about DS?" He said, "Yes, he had gone to school with a neighbor who had it." His concern wasn't the Down syndrome; rather it was where he should look to find out how to parent this child." He wasn't afraid of the DS, he didn't hesitate to have this baby with DS, and it wasn't a shock to him to be having a child with DS. It was simply a part of life, and he wanted to know how to best parent this little child who happened to have DS.

Andy's mother pondered, "If some of Andy's doctors had been around children with disabilities, or had known adults with a philosophy as above, would they have said some of the things they did? Would some of his teachers been as panicked to have him in their classes, if they had been in a childhood classroom with a child who had Down syndrome? Had I grown up with children with disabilities would I have been as shocked and lost when Andy was born?   I think not!

"Lou Brown opened our eyes and minds to the opportunities that could be ahead for Andy. Reading Robert Persky's book, <u>Circle of Friends</u>, opened our hearts to the possibilities that awaited him. His stories of children and adults with disabilities, living, going to school, and working in their communities were like shining beacons urging us on. That gleam in Andy's eyes inspired us in the beginning, and Lou Brown and Robert Persky pushed us on!

"Many others continued to illumine our path with ideas, research, writings, and presentations. I relied on my educational background to sift through research, and to evaluate what would work in the real world in our neighborhood classroom. Almost as much as the professionals with their research into best practices and educational outcomes, the anecdotal writings of parents, and of people with disabilities, continued to inspire us on our quest for what was best for Andy. And the children we came to know as Andy's friends and peers proved our hypothesis to be right; the neighborhood school was the best place in the world to prepare Andy for his future!"

Chapter 3 - The Lighthouse
Elementary School Years

Consequently, on August 28, 1990, "Who Says You Can't Change the World?" shouted from the front of a tee shirt on a small boy who got off the "regular" bus. He entered the "regular" kindergarten in Room 103 in the neighborhood school, just as his sisters and brother had before him. The planning, the meetings, the discussions of the laws were over for now.

The first President Bush had just designated the school as a Federal Blue Ribbon School, one of the highest national honors awarded a school for its programs, curriculum, discipline, and outcomes. This Blue Ribbon Honor dovetailed right in with Andy's red-letter day when he began his formal education journey at the nationally recognized school.

Andy came, letter in hand from "a little child," beginning with "The Phantom of the Opera" prelude:

Forget those wide eyed fears!
Say you'll love me, and
Anywhere you go, let me go too.
Love me, that's all I ask of you.
Want me, that's all I ask of you.

The letter continued to introduce Andy. "When I get to school, I want to do everything! I want to have the same speaking parts in programs that my classmates do. I want to go on field trips, and play music, and be on a team, and use the computer. I know I need help speaking; words are hard for me. It isn't just the sounds; it's the processing of language I have trouble with. And I need some help doing things with my hands, and I need an understanding teacher who knows that my muscles get in the way of doing things neatly. And sometimes it is really hard for me to sit in my seat for very long, and paying attention is hard. The beginnings of things are harder for me than for some. It takes me a while to get used to things, and it takes people a little while to get used to me. I hope that after we are through the beginning part, that you will want me."

Yes! Long before *inclusion* was incorporated into the jargon of every professional educator, Andy began his journey with his classmates in the class of 2003 at the school with the vision where "**everyone** is teaching and **everyone** is learning."   On that special Tuesday at the Blue Ribbon School Andy became one of the community of learners where the adults, maintaining good collaborative relationships, had already come to realize that they could not achieve their goals by acting alone, and that **everyone** was a staff developer for **everyone** else.   They soon became aware that all the while Andy struggled with reading, writing, and math along with other kindergartners he became a major force, subtly but daily, "teaching" kindness, acceptance, caring, compassion, and respect for individual differences.

The expert kindergarten teacher at the neighborhood school, Andy's first in a string of those with teacher expertise, had found that Andy liked to grind cupcakes on tables, that he didn't like art, and that he didn't like to come in from the playground. After allowing him to get himself in trouble long enough, she sat him down and demanded that he straighten up. She found that he could behave and follow the rules. From that point on she expected so much from Andy, just as she did from all her other students, that they had to give her all they had. In turn she gave them all she had, including a solid curriculum, a structured classroom where she was in charge, discipline with a loving touch which meant security for her youngsters, praise, well-timed hugs, and a belief in themselves and in each other. Most of these attributes are never found among mandated state standards; one must look under "affairs of the heart."

In that same realm, Andy's mother responded to those who asked, "How is kindergarten?" "When they said he could come, I waited for the phone call that would say they had changed their mind. But the call didn't come, and last August, he got on the bus and joined the Class of 2003. As September turned into October, I waited for a note asking me to come in and talk. I finally wrote a note asking for a conference, during which time I was told I was to have him take more responsibility for himself. 'If I didn't let him try, we would never know how far he could fly,' said his intuitive teacher, who had just stolen my lines! In November <u>my</u> thanks were that he was still at school - <u>his</u> were that he could still ride Bus No. 9 with his friends.   In December he was a star reindeer in the holiday concert, so I relaxed knowing that no one would call and ask a reindeer to find another pasture! In January he missed a lot of school because of flu, which I worried about more than a call from the school. February brought Valentine's Day, and they wouldn't break my heart then! By March I knew that he was safe for this year, as what school would demand a change for the last couple of months? By May it finally dawned on me that not only had the school professionals allowed Andy to go there - they had welcomed him. They are proud that he is there, and they have made him one of their own! How is kindergarten? It has been a wonderful year!"

Andy's mother continues, "Long after they have forgotten exactly where they learned 'the letter people,' beginning sounds, or counting to 100, long after they forget who lost their first teeth or broke their arm, this class will remember to care for and respect each other. They will view other people with compassion, and will share their unique gifts with the world, because they were carefully taught by a teacher and by her very young students."

Underscoring the fact that most behavior and beliefs are learned, "You've Got to Be Carefully Taught" was a Rodgers and Hammerstein hit from the 1949 play <u>South Pacific</u>. Portraying quite an opposite theme from these kindergarten messengers, the song of more than fifty years ago says:

> You've got to be taught to hate and fear,
> You've got to be taught from year to year.
> It's got to be drummed in your dear little ear.
> You've got to be carefully taught!
>
> You've got to be taught to be afraid
> Of people whose eyes are oddly made
> Or people whose skin is a different shade
> You've got to be carefully taught!

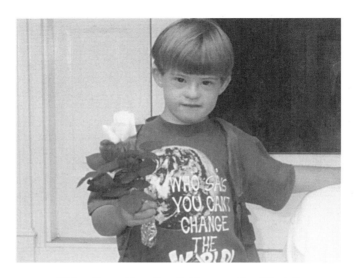

"Who Says You Can't Change the World"
shouts from Andy's shirt his
first day of kindergarten

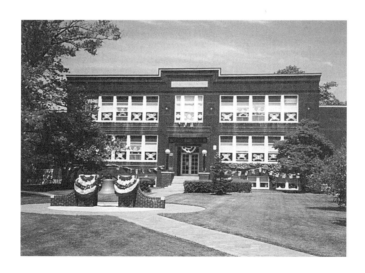

Center Street Village School
"The Lighthouse"

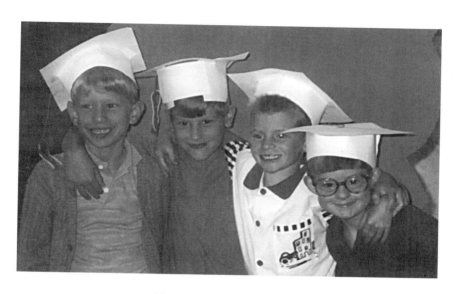

Kindergarten graduation
Buddies Paul, Derek, Johnny and Andy

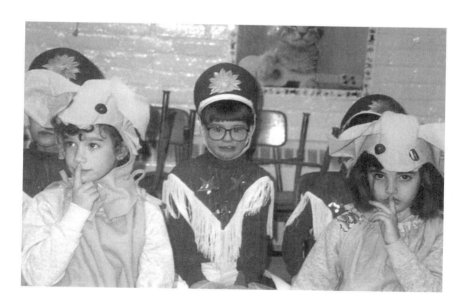

"The Nutcracker," first grade style

You've got to be taught before it's too late,
Before you are six or seven or eight
To hate all the people your relatives hate.
You've got to be carefully taught!
You've got to be carefully taught!

In the <u>Cleveland Plain Dealer</u> of May 2, 1991, Joe Dirck comments on the neighborhood school which has made Andy, a seven-year-old child with Down syndrome, one of its own. When he asked Andy's mother how it was working, she said, "It was like watching a miracle to see his development this year. He has made many new friends, and the other kids have become protective and supportive. Another success indicator was when he proudly shared his 'Student of the Month' declaration at the dinner table recently. I wrote the kindergarten teacher to thank her for giving Andy the honor. She wrote back and said, 'Andy earned this award. No thanks are necessary.'" Dirck again quotes Andy's mother, "I cried all weekend." The newspaper article was, of course, posted on the "Good News Board" at school.

Andy's first grade teacher recently emailed from her Colorado retirement home, "My experiences with Andy were a special time. I felt very privileged to have him in my class. I feel the children benefited from it, and so did I. He was a joy to have, and smiled all the time and tried very hard with his schoolwork. His mother certainly was a help with him and she was willing to do anything I asked her to do. We made a good team. I feel like he was challenged and spread his wings and flew. He worked up to his potential as far as he could and the children were always willing to help him. At first I felt nervous about having him in my class and that I could not do a good job, but he and his mother made my job a lot easier. I think by the end of the year he had accomplished a lot and we all felt very good about his first year experience. He was a special little boy and I feel good that I had some part in his elementary education."

In first grade Andy learned to read, use a number line, stay in his seat, and put his boots on alone. He learned to dance to wonderful music from <u>The Nutcracker</u>, which has become a life-long love affair. The teacher and this first grade class of youngsters had already learned that "One Size Fits All" is a myth (as anyone knows who has tried on swimsuit cover-ups recently)!

At year's end, another success indicator is the following poem from Andy to his teacher:

> If I could get my words to work, I'd have a lot to say,
> About how very grateful I am that you're my teacher every day.
> I'd tell you how exciting it is to learn to read,
> And to learn the songs you have taught me how to sing.
> And how amazed my mommy is when I can add up sums,
> And how proud my daddy is when I tell him school is fun.
> But most of all I'd like to tell how much you make me try,
> For you bring out the best in me - you urge me on that I may fly!
>
>   I love you,
>   Andy

His second grade teacher remarked, "We never know what he is going to learn, so we must try to teach him all of it." Friendships became of paramount importance in second grade also. Derek, commenting on why he was the Star of the Month, says, "I am special because I am Andy's friend." It was Derek from whom Andy received his first birthday party invitation. While Andy's parents were discussing the invitation, Dad said, with great bewilderment, "What will we do?" Mom calmly and without hesitancy said, "I suppose we'd better shop for a gift!"

One fine fall day at the beginning of Andy's third grade his mother came to the neighborhood school to speak on the topic of *Differences* to all third graders, their teachers, and the principal. During the end of her talk, she asked everyone to put a large marshmallow in his/her mouth and begin talking with one another. As all were garbling their words, she explained that this is similar to the problem that those with speech difficulties (e.g., children with Down syndrome) have in communicating. Following the excellent talk, academically-talented Sarah, who was seated next to Andy, asked "if we would know it if we met someone with differences like that?" With tears in her eyes, the thankful principal made a hasty exit from the room.

Another speech difficulty of long ago comes to mind when God called Moses to serve. He replied, "O my Lord, I am not eloquent, neither before nor since You have spoken to Your servant; but I am slow of speech and slow of tongue." "Go, and I will be with your mouth and teach you what you shall say" (Exodus 4:11-12). This language suggests that Moses may have had a speech impediment, too. Perhaps he stuttered. Often one's impairments or disabilities are used to endow people with strength and to use the limitations for good. Out of weaknesses grow courage, power, and happiness depending on faith and reliance upon Him.

The learning in the school community was further magnified that same day that Andy's mother talked to the third graders about differences. His mother winced, the principal noticed, as she spoke (privately) regarding Andy's handicap. This learned mother explained the derivation of the word *handicap*. It stems from those on city sidewalks, who with *cap* in *hand*, begged for money from passersby. The vision and understanding of the principal, among others, was greatly enhanced in the school of scholars that day!

Andy's third grade year was one of highs and lows resulting in total exercising of flexibility. His teacher's extended absences because of family illness, his own illnesses, and many other inconsistencies taught him to "go with the flow." In mid-April his mother writes to the principal: "You can save this and read it on a bad day if you like. I just want you to know what your school and all that all of you do for the children means to one little boy. We had a cardiology appointment. These sessions reduce Andy to an animal-like state, in which he is absolutely terrified. For about an hour, he had sat silently, looking only at the floor, cringing back when anyone even approached. The doctor was sure he could talk him through it, but managed only one 30-second listen before Andy started screaming.

At the second yell, the doc looked at me and said he thought we'd all been through enough for one day. He turned to Andy and asked if he wanted to be finished and go back home. 'No,' Andy replied, 'school.' The doc said okay, he was done, and that I should take him back to school.

"It was like night and day," she continued. "Andy told him all about his friends, who, he said, would be worried about him and be glad he was back, his teacher, who is very tall and very very nice, and you, the 'boss' of the school. He told the doctor about reading class with the guys, lunch, and the playground. Obviously, to Andy, school is where all the 'good stuff' is. In his life of therapy and doctors and lessons, school stands out to him as his soul, his center of all that is good and normal and 'like everyone else,' in his life. So - the good you all do - means so much!"

Andy's vision and depth of understanding were made indelible to his church community at Christmastime that year, also. Traditionally, his church incorporates the custom of families lighting the candles of the advent wreath, in addition to each family member reading designated lines regarding each candle. Andy's mother thought his part would be to name the candles, with the other family members reciting the remainder. "Sir Andrew," as his mother puts it, "would have no part in saying just four words!" After mega practicing, the little boy who brought hope, and love, and joy, and faith to a whole different level for his family and friends, told the entire congregation about these things. Candles, symbolizing the above attributes, were illumined along with the hearts of the churchgoers on that Christmas Eve of 1994.

The early primary grades were now behind Andy, with the help of occupational and speech therapists, his daily tutor who adapted (often rewrote) the curriculum, and his "North Star" mother. A big change in the fourth grade was the advanced curriculum; additionally, the classroom was physically upstairs. Fire drills were truly a test for Andy. If it was a "planned" drill he was always previously forewarned because he could not tolerate the fierce sound of the fire bell (earplugs were used). If the alarm was accidentally pushed, it was extremely unpleasant for Andy, his classmates and teacher. The steep stairs (vintage 1914) were not easy on his little legs encased in braces either. The principal realized that Andy was truly "one of the gang," upon investigating the unusually long building evacuation time during the initial fire drill at the beginning of his fourth grade. The principal was overwhelmed when she finally determined the reason for this extended evacuation time. She discovered that every one of his classmates was taking one stair at a time, clumping down and clumping back up, because that's the only way Andy could conquer the old steep stairs. To add to her very emotional visual were the reflector lights blinking on and off from the back of many fourth-graders' tennis shoes which many students wore. Clump, clump, blink, blink, clump . . . remains an indelible visual and audible Kodak moment in her mind!

Additionally, fourth grade was a year of tremendous growth and accomplishment. After a week with a wonderful teacher, a substitute had to be called in for the entire first semester. Her first assignment out of college, the "sub" believed that if a child was in her class, she must teach him. She got busy right away teaching and holding high expectations for **everyone** in her class. She taught Andy how to take written tests, to multiply, to write down his thoughts, just as his other classmates.

Perhaps Nick Lyons was right when he said, "The way to teach Andy stuff is to do it with one of us." Nick already knew, by the fourth grade, how to engineer and operate the well-worn phrase, "good teaching is good teaching."

Andy's peers continued to befriend him, both in the classroom academically and outside socially. The social "coolness" which every child must have to "fit in" became a very important issue with Andy. His mother comments, "Although I always knew with our other children that it was important for them to feel that they fit in with their friends, I also knew that it was up to me to teach them to be themselves. I always made it clear that I could not worry about what everyone else did, or what they had, or what they were allowed to do . . . I was only concerned about them!

"So why is it that this summer I am possessed with nine-year-old boys, and what is cool to them?   Suddenly it seems more important to have Andy be cool than it ever mattered with the other children.   Perhaps what set me off was an incident at Andy's class picnic, when for the first time, I saw children in Andy's grade be really mean to one another.

"Andy was fine, and just one of the kids.   But another little boy wasn't. He was on a team, and no one wanted to stand by him.   Some of the kids teased him for running the way he did, for his squeaky voice, for his shoes.   I was appalled.   It was my game to organize.   I laid down the law that they were on the team they were on, and if they didn't want to be on that team, and stand where their place was, they could sit on the grass and not be a part of what we were doing.   No one took me up on the offer to quit playing, and the remarks stopped.   But then the child was just ignored. He is a 'regular' kid, as far as I know.   But he is a child who stands out from the rest.   He simply is not attuned to the things the others are.   His clothes, conversation topics, his mannerisms are all a bit different, and it is just enough to make him definitely not cool.

"These same children seem to welcome Andy, who as we all know, has his own set of differences.   I think, that because Andy's differences have a name, that perhaps it is easier for the kids to understand the whys and ways of Andy.   But I also know the effort that has been made to assure that Andy is as cool as he can be.   The clothes, the haircut make the first impression, so I watch intensively what the others wear and how they cut their hair.   This is easy enough for me to do.   But recently, coolness has become more complicated.   Coolness caused me to wander around 'Toys R Us' recently trying to decide for a long time, whether I should buy a 'Super Shooter' for him or not.   I don't buy guns, and since this was for a religious holiday present, I really was in a bind.   Everyone else on the street has water guns.   I knew that he would want to play with them this summer, and if he didn't have one, he either could watch them on the sidelines, or use something else and be different.   The 'Super Shooter' won out.

"And then there was the discussion with Andy, in the grocery aisle about what we would get for the baseball team snacks. First, I tried for real juice drinks, sort of knowing that he would nix that idea. Juice boxes were also on the nix list, in addition to the bottles that were on sale that day. I knew that the 'Squeezits' were the coolest of cool. He knew it too, and so the few cents that I would have saved on the sale bottles was just not worth it. He wanted the cool stuff to pass out to the team! And now, in the name of coolness, Andy's lunch sandwiches must be cut into two pieces, instead of the more manageable, but babyish, four. For the sake of coolness, big sis Megan gives him his last-minute instructions at baseball games. It is definitely <u>not</u> cool to have Mom or Dad talk to their player on the bench!

"All the coolness issues were not as easy as these. These I can chalk up to growing pains (on both our parts). But I also want him to speak with his friends as a cool kid, and that the topics will be age appropriate even if the sentence structure isn't. I want him to read books that tell nine-year-old stories, even if they are simple to read. I want him to learn to do a job that other children his age are doing, even if he takes twice as long to do it.

"I learned a lesson at that picnic. It's cool to be different, if you are cool in other ways, too. But if you are only different, it isn't cool at all!"

Andy's mother created a "cool" poem to celebrate Andy's tenth birthday:

Hallelujah! The boy is ten!
What a world of difference between now and then!

It was a day in February, breezy and warm
When, hallelujah! The boy was born.
A cute little thing, ten fingers and toes,
But something was wrong, so the story goes.

They took him away in the dead of night
Looked him all over to see what was right,
The heart wasn't working, so they found,
And later, they added, he might have Downs.

The doctors tested, and poked, and probed,
They treated, and patched, and then they sewed.
They fixed what they could for the little boy,
And then they said, "Relax, sit back, and enjoy!"

Next the therapists and teachers got their turn,
They taught him what they could get him to learn.
Movement, and talking, buttons and pins,
There was even one to teach him to swim.

Finally, as ready as he could be,
He entered kindergarten, in room 103.
Cutting and pasting, and letters, and then,
Recess, and time to play with his FRIENDS!

The years have gone quickly, too fast it seems,
And my baby exists now only in dreams,
The boy that I have is now tall and thin,
And enters a room like a whirling wind!

He says to me, over and over again,
Can you believe it, Mom? I am ten!
Yes, miracles happen, and things do work out,
My boy is ten now, I quietly shout . . .

Hallelujah! The boy is ten!
What a world of difference between now and then!

A highlight that year was the commemoration of the 50th Anniversary of World War II by the entire 350-student body at the school. The celebration was the culmination of a month-long study on wars involving the United States. The Keynote Speaker, Rep. Steven C. LaTourette (R-OH), spoke about Memorial Day, Patriotism, and World War II to the students, teachers, parents, and many WW II grandfather veterans who were the honored guests for the all-day event. If any veteran present that day had a remaining doubt why they suffered and fought in the violence of World War II fifty years ago, it was erased as they were escorted to the stage hand in hand with their grandchildren ambassadors.   In the Cleveland Plain Dealer the next day, April McClellan-Copeland reported: "Fourth graders Nick Meyer, Andy Patterson, and Paul Markell are like any other schoolboys - they like sports, and wear oversized Cleveland Indians and Chicago Bulls jerseys. But when it came time for the trio to stand before veterans at a Memorial Day ceremony yesterday and recite the World War I poem, 'In Flanders Fields,' the boys displayed solemnity and patriotism far beyond their years." A 21-gun salute and taps closed the day's ceremonies. One cannot help remembering the sacrifices made by these veterans in order that freedom can be celebrated, in order that three fourth graders (one of whom has language difficulties) can "display solemnity and patriotism far beyond their years as they recite the John McCrae poem," bridging a two-generation gap.   How proud Andy's veteran Grandfather (now deceased) would have been to be escorted to center stage by his grandchild, along with all the other veterans who were honored!   How proud he would have been to hear Andy recite "In Flanders Fields" with his buddies.

Lieutenant Colonel John McCrae, MD, would also be proud that his poem was being recited by these young orators exactly 70 years after it was first published in "Punch" in London in 1915.

IN FLANDERS FIELDS the poppies blow
Between the crosses, row on row,
That mark our place, and in the sky
The larks, still bravely singing, fly
Scarce heard amid the guns below.

We are the Dead. Short days ago
We lived, felt dawn, saw sunset glow,
Loved and were loved, and now we lie
in Flanders fields.

Take up our quarrel with the foe:
To you from failing hands we throw
The torch; be yours to hold it high.
If ye break faith with us who die
We shall not sleep. Though poppies grow
in Flanders fields.

One of the most memorable poems ever written, McCrae composed the verse in the back of an ambulance parked near the dressing station just a few hundred yards north of the Belgium city of Ypres. He wrote as a vent for his anguish about the death of a young friend and former student who was killed by a shell burst. Although McCrae had served as a doctor in the South African War, he felt it impossible to get used to the suffering, the screams, and the blood at Ypres.

Andy's mother felt a much different type of suffering when shortly after knowing that she had given birth to a boy and thinking, "I'll be going to baseball games forever," she was advised to add baseball to the list of things her newborn would never do. However six years later, as Andy himself had erased several things on his "would never do" list through his own determination, Mom saw that he was playing baseball with some of the neighborhood children. He told her he learned it in gym; and "Sure!" he would like to be on a team and play with his friends when his sister later asked him (without asking mother first). The man whom mom asked if they would allow a little boy with Down syndrome to play on the team surprised her when he said, "If the boy wants to play baseball, he should play baseball."

"The boy," Andy, was paired with a coach who was not content to have him sit on the bench, but taught him to hit, and to catch, and to play the right field position. Whenever the coach worked with a small group on basic skills, Andy was there. He listened and he learned. Time and again - "Watch the ball!" Time and again - "pay attention!" Time and again - "Watch the batter!" Time and again - (quietly from mother) - "Don't let the ball hurt him!" Time and again - "Don't let him mess up!"

Barbara Davis

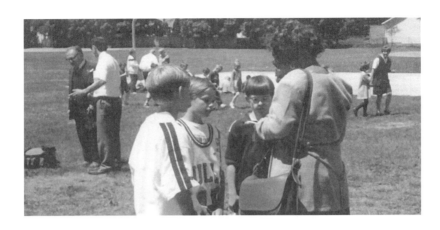

April McClellen-Copeland of the "Cleveland Plain Dealer" interviews Patriots
Paul, Nick and Andy – May 26, 1995

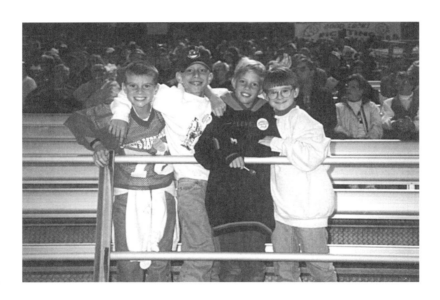

Friday night football in Mentor
Pals Johnny, Paul, Nick and Andy

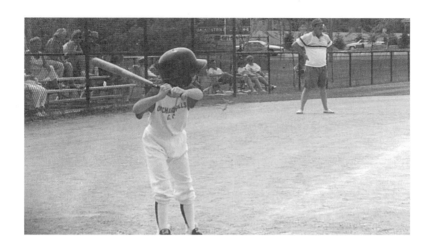

Hey batta, batta, batta!

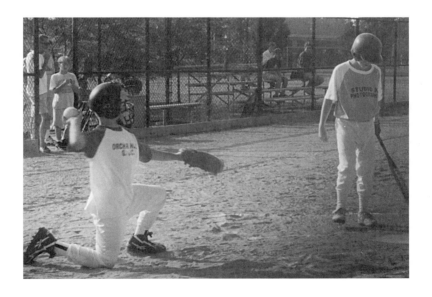

. . . And a fine catcher at that!

He did turn out to be a good hitter. Getting on the batting helmet was hard with his glasses, and his stance was awkward, and some of his "hits" were due to the inexperience of the fielders, but it was a thrill to have bat meet ball at this stage. The team lost more games than they won, and tied a few that they didn't lose. When they did win, the parents were ecstatic, too.

During a post-season conversation with Andy's parents, the coach related that at the beginning of the season, the coaches were told that a child with a disability wanted to play. "Does anybody want him?" There had been a silence, but a new coach thought if a child wanted to play he should have the chance. He said the big YES word! Andy's mother reflects, "We would all live happily ever after if there were more people like the new coach who saw a little boy who just wanted to play a game and who was willing to do what needed to be done to make the game worth playing. I learned a lot that season, also," she continued, "I no longer list the things the boy will never do. Time has a way of changing things."

The following season began with another coach, new teammates, and new challenges. "Right field is 'our' position and we are proud!" And mother is thankful not too many balls are hit sharply there, assuring relative safety. She is also thankful not to have a pitcher son. She explains, "When you are a kid and you are good, parents sometimes forget that you are just a kid. But my kid's sole claim to fame is that he is a part of the team. As the season wore on, the ball did get hit to right field a few times, and most of the time Andy fielded it, and threw it in.

"How he loves it! There is the uniform, the snacks, the coaches (who have really taught him about playing and have been kind and encouraging, and a little demanding all at once); and there is the male bonding. Baseball noises don't have to be made clearly to be understood. He quickly learned to join the other players who yell 'hey, batta, batta, batta' at the top of their lungs. He quickly learned to slap backs, pull down caps, and wear his cap backwards. He also learned to toe the dirt at the plate when he is at bat, glaring at the opposing pitcher as if he hits a homer every time. What he lacks in strength and coordination, he compensates for in heart." He began to hit the ball – first they were foul tips, then pop-ups, but the contact was there. Finally came the night when he smashed it, and the ball went up the middle for an honest base hit. He actually scored a run, and the team won the game. Victory was as sweet as the ice cream, topped by the coach's presentation of the game ball to Andy, signed by every player and coach. Does life get any better for an eight-year-old boy?" Jackie Gleason said it first, "How sweet it is!" Andy and team applied it!

Each season usually starts with a few parents and a few children looking sideways at Andy. His mother says, "You can read their minds as they wonder what he is doing on their team. And every season part way through, one feels the groundswell of good thoughts going with him as he walks to the plate. And each season there is finally the time he walks, or hits, and gets on base, and the parents cheer as if he had hit a home run. And when he makes it all around to score a run, every player on the team 'high fives' him. And we let out a collective breath. . .and he sits down, trying to look as if he had done this every day!"

Andy's mother comments about baseball. "It's real, ten-year-old life to be on a team. Baseball is being hot and sweaty, getting your clothes covered with the field, and dripping the post-game chocolate ice cream over it all. It is learning to revel in the moments of triumph - a catch, a hit, a victory, a walk - and that the definition of triumph depends on who is defining it. It is learning to accept the called third strike, the missed ball, and the short end of the score - and the short end of the score means different things to different people. And it's learning that a good team sticks together and cares about one another, no matter what. Being on a team, being a real part of it, means caring for the player whether he hits the homer or strikes out, if he pitches the shutout or throws the gopher ball, if he makes the great catch, or drops the ball. You tell teammates to wait till next time. You tell them it was the trying that counts and theirs was a great try. My boy needs to know all that. So do the other 13 players on the team. So do we all."

Andy's mother reports on the third game of the next season - the top of the third inning! "While I saw the 'safe' in right field, Andy had other aspirations; he yearned to play shortstop and he asked the coach in practice if he might play there. He talked about wanting that position, and I should have known what was coming. When we were at bat, we began to catch up to the other team. Excitement churned on our side of the field. If only we could keep them from scoring we had a chance to come back and win the game. Our team was taking their positions on the field, when Andy ran over to say that he was going to change positions - to shortstop! I said no, he wasn't! I told him that he couldn't, that he would be killed, as I tried to signal the coach! Andy ran out to the infield. My 'safe' right fielder became the shortstop, I couldn't watch! I couldn't not watch! I was sure he would be hurt, or would at least miss the plays and lose the game. Out on the infield, Andy was a model of attention. He assumed the ready position, and never took his eyes off the batters or the balls. The first batter struck out, and I breathed a sigh of relief. 'You better be ready!' I shouted as the next batter stood in and popped to the pitcher. 'Get set out there!' I yelled as the third kid approached the plate. He lined the ball straight out to right field, where the right fielder caught it to retire the side. Andy trotted in, looking at us with the I-took-care-of-things look on his face. They finished the game with Andy back in right field. He stood taller, and paid attention. And then in our last at bat, he smacked a hit with two outs, to keep their rally going! Andy scored the tying run of the game, and we went on to win! Wow! It is enough for me that he is able to be a part of a team; that he can experience the fun of the uniforms, practices, and after-game treats. When he connects with the ball, it is a bonus. When no one catches the ball he has hit, I am thrilled!"

Andy's mother calls this game a "career highlight!" She continues, "To see how he reacted to the challenge the coach offered him, reminded me that 'quiet, safe, and boring' is not always best. That if we are never challenged, we cannot grow. That if we cannot try, we would never know what might have been. To see the other boys on the team simply accept that Andy was the shortstop for that inning, to hear them cheer him on when he was up to bat, made me realize that sometimes gusto and determination will get you through, even though you might not be really ready to take the next step. I have read that baseball imitates life. I know that the lessons learned on the field tend to stay with the boys long after the game is over. Those 12 little boys saw how much it meant for Andy to have a chance to play the position he dreamed of. They saw him play better than they, or he, knew he could, when 'quiet, safe, and boring' was replaced by a real challenge. They learned about encouraging a teammate. They learned that it makes everyone feel good, to give someone a chance. And they learned that there are times in life when you have to play a little harder yourself, to be sure all the bases are covered."

At some point every child has a coach that <u>must</u> win! Andy was no exception. His next season coach wanted to win. He did not yell, he did not berate his players, but he did want to win. He treated all the boys fairly, but he did want to win. In the draft that was held in the spring to assign players to a   team who were new to the league, he wanted players who could help his team win. He didn't know Andy. The coach who wanted to win, chose Andy - certainly not because of his reputation as a star player.

When the coach who wanted to win called to introduce himself and give the practice schedule, he was quick to say that his team last year had been good, very good, and that many of those boys would be back this year. At the first practice, Andy's family realized the boys were not only good, they were big, very big. Eddie, the coach's son, was over six feet tall, and built with a powerful body and long legs. The coach decided that Andy should be the catcher. No more could he day dream out in right field; no more could he kick at the grass, bat at the bugs with his hat, and watch the game from afar. The coach worried that in this league, the kids could place their hits there, and Andy would get hurt by their sharp line drives. Andy was delighted with his new position! Before the constant catch, stand, throw, squat would take their toll at some point, in most games he looked good. Andy's mother prayed a lot! She prayed that the batter would remember who was right behind him, that Andy would not stand up in that fraction of a second when the bat was coming around, and that he would not lose the game for the team on a close play at the plate.

As the season got into full tilt, it became more and more apparent that the coach who wanted to win had known what he was doing when he picked Andy.   The team was a better team because he was part of it.   While

Eddie was hitting all of his homers and racing around the bases, Mark was pitching the team out of jams, Ryan was throwing them out at first, and Eric was doing his acrobatics in the field and around the bases, Andy was making them all play on a higher level. Since they knew Andy would not catch a hurried throw to the plate, they had to catch the fly balls and throw in carefully, and get the other team out before they were running to home. They had to get those ground balls, and make the plays on the bases. The pitcher knew that he had to back up the plate on any close play, and they all knew, that if they were up and Andy was on base, he needed them to either homer, or walk so he would have a chance to score! He played better too, being with them. His teammates gave him advice, told him to hustle, handed him his mask, told him to get the pop-ups, to retrieve the foul balls, all encased in kindness.

"As Andy learned baseball from the boys, they learned life from him," observes Andy's mother. "Encouragement helps. Keep trying. Success feels good. Get to first base any way you can. Everyone counts. Play hard. Hard is different for everyone. In the great scheme of things, a dropped ball just isn't that important. Ice cream is a great equalizer. Life is worth whatever it takes to really live it."

She continued, "Tournament Day was the kind of hot summer day that just begged for boys to be on the baseball diamond, and the team had an excellent won/lost record. The first time Andy was up, he hit the ball, and the kid fumbled it, and he reached first base. A walk allowed him second base, and a powerful hit beyond the outfielders allowed him to score . . . and there was joy in Mudville! The next time he got up, he also reached first safely. Flushed by his first success, he was determined to score, but the fates didn't allow it. The next player hit a grounder, and Andy was out at second. In his excitement, he didn't hear the ump call him out, and the coach had to call over to him to tell him to go sit down. His chin dropped, and he trudged off and into the dugout. His teammates greeted him with pats and high fives, and told him it had been a great hit, that there was nothing he could have done to be safe at second, and that he'd get it next time. At that moment, not one of those boys cared about the score, or that Andy was out - they just cared about their teammate who had tried so hard, and done his best, and felt so bad! I was biting my lip watching, figuring no one would understand if the tears spilled over, when one of the moms loudly yelled, 'And they say that there aren't any good kids in the world! Look at those boys!' She was so proud of them, proud not of their baseball ability, but of the way they were treating one small boy who so very much wanted to be one of them! It became clear that, although the championship would not be determined until later, that these boys were true champions in all of our hearts.

"The game went on, of course, and even though the best team does not always win, on this day, it did. We won that game, and in the third and last game of the tournament, we became the Champions!" Andy's mother exclaimed, "Andy hit in that game, too, and scored! The look on his face, and on the faces of the team members when they greeted him in the dugout, will forever be etched in my heart. Some moms get to see their sons hit homeruns, or get an MVP trophy, or win a scholarship, or become a professional athlete. Well this was *my* moment to watch my Champion, and sweet it was!

"Dad and I talked later in the night, still a little surprised at the way things had turned out, that the coach who wanted to win, had won, not in spite of having Andy on the team, but because of the way the team had come together as a team. The team became cohesive by helping each other, covering for each other, and caring for and encouraging each other. And we talked of the boy who had said he was faster and stronger and could play with the big boys, and how hard he had tried, and how he had proven himself right." Yes! One is reminded of Henry Ford's saying, "Whether you think you can, or you think you can't, you are probably right!"

The season is over, and Andy will go on to another league next year, if there is next year for him to play ball. Andy's mother was again in a state of dismay: "Yesterday, I asked him if he thought he would like to play softball again next year. His answer was immediate. 'No, I am not.' A little surprised, I asked, 'Why?' In a tone that let me know he had thought it all over, he answered, 'Because I am going to play hardball!' He very definitely will not play hardball - but I am a bit worried, because he had the same expression on his face as he did when he informed us that he was going to play shortstop!"

Academically, Andy continued to march to his own drum during the fifth and sixth grades at the school with the vision and the mission to educate **everyone**. Fifth grade was projects, and Andy loved them. He found that making things was a new way to learn. He found that he was a real part of a real world; he grew in many ways, not only academically, but emotionally and physically as well. One of Andy's highlights of the year was the springtime "growing up unit," complete with the gift of deodorant!

All sixth graders go to camp every year as a part of their school experience. Parents are often reluctant to send their young students off for a full week on their own - many for the very first time. Andy's mother was, of course, on this list. Anxious is an understated word for feelings to describe both mother and teachers, as each worried about different things. "My worries are the usual mother things, heightened to a degree by Andy's unique challenges. Theirs center on him falling, being injured, or having a very hard time doing some of the activities. The gorge walk is a major concern; the path is steep and narrow, they worry about him going down and coming up. I worry that he will get lost as he wanders around at the bottom. So, of course, we have had meetings.

"True to form, Andy has not worried about camp. He didn't come to the meetings. He has talked about it very little, until one day last week. We were doing errands. The car has always been one of the best places for a good talk, so I started talking camp. Mostly, I told him that it sounded so exciting that I wanted to go, too. Of course, he said that I couldn't. (Little did he know he had the school district policy backing him!)

> "Camp sounds like so much fun, I want to got too!"
> "You can't."
> "But I want to."
> "No, mom."
> "Maybe I could go as a helper."

"No."

"But, please! I could help the teachers! I could cook!"

"NO!"

"But what if you need me?"

"I won't."

"But what if you go on a hike and get lost?"

"I'll have to find my way back."

"But what if you fall in the mud and get all wet?"

"I'll go to my cabin."

"But what if you go on the boat, and it tips?"

"Then I'll swim!"

"But what if you go on a walk on a steep hill and you get scared and it's too hard?"

"Then maybe I'll fall."

"And then what will you do?"

"Then, mom, I'll just have to get up!"

"I had no further questions. I swallowed my pride, admitted to myself that I had been out-thought by a little kid who is not supposed to be able to think too well. I swallowed my hurt at being left behind, and turned into the shoe store. We got him his pair of hiking boots. He'll need them when he goes on the gorge walk with his class."

The following is an ironic epilogue to the hiking boots. The day of the gorge walk dawned clear, following three days of heavy rain. The hiking boots were new and ready to go, but had quickly become favorites of the little kid. Heaven forbid that they should get any spots of mud on them. On his own and without suggestions from anyone, Andy decided to wear his loose-fitting, rubber boots (with no support) on the gorge walk. He not only managed the walk just fine, he was selected to be the leader and the pacesetter! As he was the only one with waterproof boots on, he was the only one allowed to go wading in the stream when they reached the bottom of the gorge.

The last "chapter" on camping came much later when Andy's mother learned what a wonderful week it was, as he told her about the gorge walk, wading in the creek, boating, the dance, the cabin – all of it! Much later she learned other "details" of camp. It seems that a child from their partner school was tormenting Andy every chance he got. Andy's friends took it for two days, and then took matters into their own hands. The boys from school, all trained in techniques of walking away from confrontation, of going to adults if there were problems, of mediating their disputes, confronted the offender. They made sure (it was better that few adults, including Andy's family and the school personnel, never learned quite how) that this child would never again treat Andy badly. This action was done at a huge risk, for when one goes to camp, any hint of trouble is reason to be sent home. But, you see, Andy is their friend, and they did for him, what boys do for friends. Andy's mother, in retelling what she knew of the incident, said, "The boys drew their line in the sand, and stood up for what was right. Bless them, every one!"

This is the school where parents and students often teach each other and "the professionals" about learning, and more importantly, about living. This is the school where teachers and leaders have made the commitment to educate **everyone**, even those born with the "regular" twenty-three pairs of chromosomes (determining hair color, eye color, height, etc.) in addition to those students with an extra chromosome which causes Down syndrome.

In addition to the school's commitment to teach **everyone**, Andy's mother does not limit her concerns to her son, but is an advocate for others with disabilities and psychological disorders. For example, she was compelled to "educate" a professional (privately in writing) when he publicly implied that the parents of a young adolescent (who was suspended from school) "*found* a psychologist who pronounces that their son is a victim of a specific disorder." In her letter to the orator, she said, "No parent wants their child labeled as having such a disorder if it can be avoided. These labels, these diagnoses, follow children their whole life, and are not something parents seek to have so that their child's behavior will be excused. The diagnosis of any behavioral disorder is a very sensitive issue because of attitudes exactly like that which you displayed to your audience - while smirking, if only they would have been better parents, their child would not be in this difficulty." She concludes with a powerful query, "Can people with clinical depression help having the depression?" Case closed.

Another benchmark demonstrating compassion and advocacy for others was the founding of "The Upside of Downs," by Andy's parents in 1987. His mother often contributed to the organization's *Newsletter.* She explains her rationale and the parent group's philosophy. "When the fires of passion run on low, and we are tired of always having to be 'The Ones,' the strength comes from the other parents in our group who understand. For we have found, in the group, that joy when shared is multiplied, that worry shared is divided, and that hope shared burns ever brighter. May all of us inspire each other on this journey we share!" Robert Fulghum says it in his book, <u>All I Really Need to Know I Learned in Kindergarten,</u> as he explains one of his basic premises, "We need to hold hands and stick together!"

Andy's birthday his "senior year" at the elementary school is recorded by his mother as "more than a celebration of Andy's birth and life. It is a celebration of hope fulfilled, prayers answered, and love personified in each and every one of our lives." She reminisces about that long, dark night thirteen years ago when the baby was born. "My joy and happiness vanished! I cried, and I worried. I was terrified by the thoughts that went through my head. I cried for the baby, for the kids, for his father, and for me. Slowly, the healing began, and our family found that life not only goes on, it gets better."

It got better for his grandparents who lived just long enough to "know we were heading in the general direction of being all right." It got better for his younger sister, Megan, who was his advocate. (He has her big brown eyes.) She has written beautiful essays about her life with Andy, and used them for her college applications, so that people will have no doubt as to who she is - and who he is. His older sister, Speech Therapist Katie, is a cheerleader for all her clients, just as she always has been for Andy.

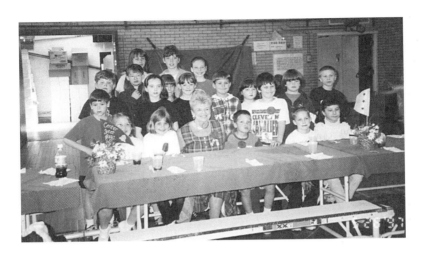

Waiting for pizza at Patriots' Lunch

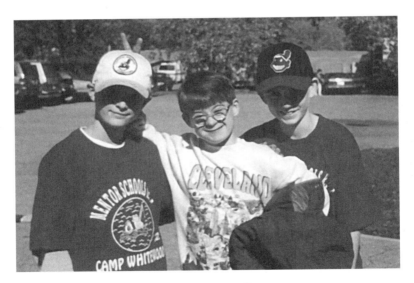

WJ, Andy and Phil return safely from 6th grade Camp Whitewood

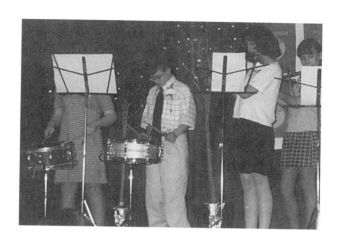

Drummer boy during graduation

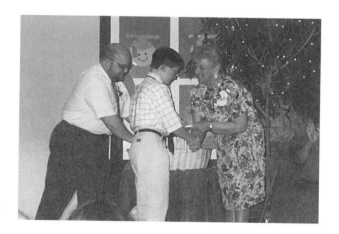

"The Moment"
Andy receives his diploma from Teacher
David Porter and Principal Barbara Davis

(He is practical, just like Katie.) And it got better for his older brother, Boomer, who was a little chagrined at 12 years-of-age that his parents were having a baby, and worse yet, a baby like Andy. (He has his hands.) Years later he proudly announced that he chose Andy to be his "Best Man" at his wedding. When someone questioned if he could do it, Boomer looked a little puzzled and a little hurt, "I just always thought I would have Andy!" Yes, life continues to get better for his family and for him, the boy with his dad's sense of humor and his mom's love of books.

Another genre of books was the customary <u>Memory Book</u> created and produced by the sixth grade graduating class each year at the neighborhood school. One of the traditional questions posed to members of the class was, "Who do you most admire and why?" Predictably, most answered with the rich and famous; i.e., Albert Einstein, Michael Jordon, Thomas Edison, Sandy Alomar, Nelson Mandela. In this author's opinion, however, the highlight was the reply of Sean who wrote, "I admire Andy Patterson because he is successful in school even with Down syndrome."

Pioneer Andy, always in regular classes, was proud of himself as he graduated from his school of choice June 4th, 1997. He made his family proud during his struggles and triumphs; the members of the staff, his class and their families also took great pride in his accomplishments. His teacher, David Porter, prefaces Andy's approach to the stage: "We have all had the opportunity to watch one young man overcome the odds and be a successful student."

With applause bouncing off the walls of the auditorium for Andy, the principal appeared to have a problem with her eyes when she proudly presented the diplomas that year. The personnel in the school with the vision that **everyone** is teaching and **everyone** is learning had all fallen under Andy's spell!

This spring of '97 heralded "graduation time," and retirement, for the principal of the school with the vision. She presented a golden acorn pin engraved with the words, **"Together We Made Differences,"** to each staff member as a farewell remembrance to all the courageous people who were unafraid to think out of the box. Attached to each acorn was the verse:

> **The acorn symbolizes the seeds we sowed,**
> **At the school with colors of blue and gold.**
> **May our paths of excellence continue,**
> **Illumined by friendship and a rainbow hue.**

"Paths of excellence" were also heralded for the past seven years by Andy's mother. She writes to the talented, creative, and giving staff, "He can now zip, tie, button, snap, read, write, add, subtract, multiply, and divide. He can share his thoughts, and hopes, and dreams with anyone who will listen. He can shoot baskets, hit a ball, catch a pass. He can do a thousand other things, all because of all of you in the village!" She includes in that school village, the classroom teachers, the tutors and aids, the nurse, the custodian, lunch staff, playground supervisors, the music, gym, and art teachers, the librarian, secretary, and the principal. She thanks all who helped him with each step, from learning how to teach him what he needed to know, getting the stones out of his braces, enlarging music as he became a percussionist, telephoning, and to coming in off the playground. Yes, it takes a village to raise a child! It also takes devoted parents who will communicate his needs to others if he is unable, who will work with him as he does his homework night after night, who will inspire and contribute to his projects, and all the while - believing, achieving, and succeeding together.

The seeds of success were also recorded by Andy's mother in a video of his school activities, achievements, and accomplishments. She selected the dynamic lyrics and music, "Standing Outside the Fire," by Garth Brooks as accompaniment. The words of the perfect merger of talent and truth follow:

> We call them cool, those hearts that have no scars to show,
> The ones that never do let go, and risk the tables being turned.

We call them fools, who have to dance within the flame,
Who chance the sorrow and the shame, that always comes with
    getting burned.
But you've got to be tough when consumed by desire,
'Cause it's not enough just to stand outside the fire.
We call them strong, those who can face this world alone,
Who seem to get by on their own, those who will never take
    the fall.
We call them weak, who are unable to resist,
The slightest chance love might exist, and for that forsake it all.
They're so hell-bent on giving, walking a wire,
Convinced it's not living if you stand outside the fire.
Standing outside the fire, standing outside the fire,
Life is not tried, it is merely survived, if you're standing outside
    the fire.
Standing outside the fire, standing outside the fire,
There's this love that is burning deep in my soul,
Constantly yearning to get out of control,
Wanting to fly higher and higher, I can't abide standing outside
    the fire.
Life is not tried, it is merely survived, if you're standing outside
    the fire.

It was at this time that Andy expressed the desire that his ashes be connected somehow with the school. "Life is not tried, it is merely survived, if you're standing outside the fire. . . "

Andy and his family again understood that "Life is not tried, it is merely survived, if you're standing outside the fire." They understood "the love that is burning deep in my soul, constantly yearning to get out of control. . . . . .I can't abide standing outside the fire." The circle of life - of understanding - was completed when Andy's namesake, Aunt Andrea (one of the rare people who sees him as just a kid who happened to be her nephew and not a kid with Down syndrome) was hospitalized. Andy sensed by the tone and conversations in the house that it was serious. Suddenly as the family was getting ready to visit her, with telling eyes

Andy asked if this sickness of Auntie's was serious? They were shocked as they realized in that very moment a circle had been completed! The love and support that Auntie has always given, was about to come right back to her, not just from the adults, but from the one who had needed so much of it. "I stood as I watched the changing of the guard, the passing of the torch, the circle of love being completed before our very (tearful) eyes!" relates Andy's mother.

"A ship in a port is safe, but that is not what ships are built for" (Admiral Grace Hopper). These words capture the rough and windy journey to junior high school for Andy. One of the paramount worries for his family was that his steadfast elementary school friends, with their own adolescent fears and desires of fitting in and staying "cool," might abandon Andy. A friend was amazed that the family, who most usually used good straight thinking, would think that. They gently reminded them of the camp "incident" when no parents, teachers, nor counselors knew there was a problem. They could have walked away then, among <u>many</u> other times!

It seems noteworthy here to quote the dedication in Child Psychologist Sylvia Rimm's book, <u>Exploring Feelings</u>. She says: "Dedicated to the caring parents and teachers who share the stresses and the joys of guiding adolescents toward a fulfilling adult life." The irony is that <u>Exploring Feelings</u> is a discussion book for <u>Gifted Kids Have Feelings Too.</u> No! One size *never* fits all!

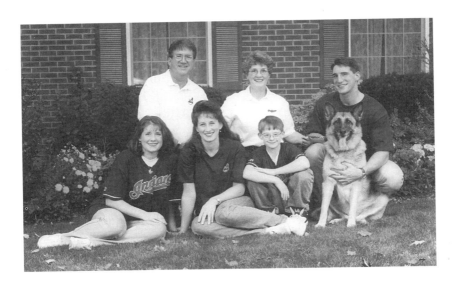

Tom, Paula and Boomer Patterson
Megan, Katie, Andy and Masie

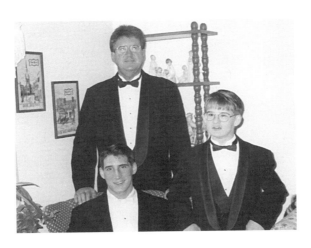

Patterson men at Boomer's wedding
September 20, 1997

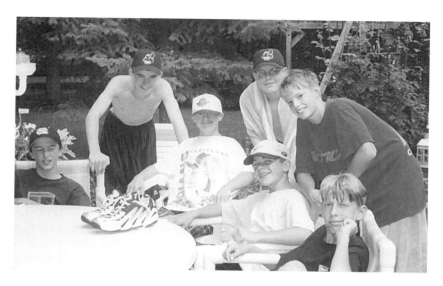

Buddies in the good 'ole summer time
WJ, Phil, Andy, Jagger, Dan, Nick and Paul

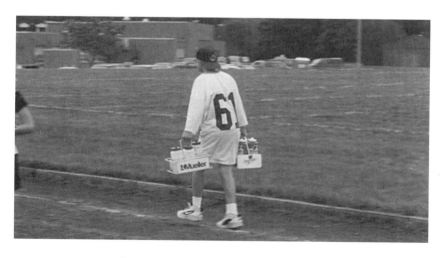

8th grade trainer Andy at Ridge Jr. High

Chapter 4 - Arctic Storm
Junior High School Years

The next what-appeared-to-be a tidal wave was the junior high administration who believed Andy would fare better in the special classes designed for those with disabilities. After much in-depth perseverance, Andy's mother (and others) finally convinced the professionals that Andy learned best in regular classes with his friends and not in the "special programs" where they thought he would benefit. Among "the others" mentioned above was a group of parents who, on August 22, 1997, wrote and signed an eloquent letter addressed to the junior high principal:

We all attended the 7th grade Orientation Program, and we felt very welcomed by the comments made by all the speakers. What we heard was how important it is to be involved in your child's school and education. The atmosphere that evening was one of caring, warmth, and cooperation. You presented an understanding that the transition to seventh grade, and junior high, can be scary, but that you and your staff would be there to help in any way possible.

We would like to tell you about a very wonderful boy and his amazing family, and how they have affected the lives of so many. When our children entered kindergarten with Andy (Patterson), many of us were wary of how his presence would impact our children. Little did we know at the time the valuable gifts that he would eventually share with us. He has helped us parents teach our children some of life's most valuable lessons: Help each other, differences can be good, look for similarities, we're more alike than we are different, cooperate with each other, work as a team, share, be kind to each other, be loyal to your friends, watch out for each other, be honest with each other. His family has also had a tremendous impact on all of us. They are parents who strive to provide the best possible life for their child. Could they possibly do any less? Because our children have been taught to be concerned and help each other, they are all very unnerved about the situation Andy is now facing. It's scary for all of our children to attend a new school, change classes for the first time, meet a lot of new students and be accepted, worry about opening a locker, etc. When they think about Andy being assigned to 'special' classes, having to face all of it without any of them there, they become very upset. When a couple of us spoke to the guidance counselors, we were told that this was the 'real world,' that everything would work out – in other words – butt out! First of all that goes against everything that was said the night of Orientation when we were encouraged to share our concerns, that our input was valuable, to expect full cooperation, and to get involved in our child's school. We also believe that the 'real world' is NOT cold, heartless, uncaring, and uncompromising, and that is what we have taught our children. People care for each other and help each other in the 'real world,' and we certainly hope your school won't teach them otherwise. To some of us who are new to your school, this unwillingness to change Andy's 'special' schedule appears to be an attempt to punish him for some reason – to set him up to fail. We find this very disconcerting and, frankly, alarming. We heard one thing at the Orientation, but are witnessing what we consider to be the opposite. It makes all of us, parents and students, much more apprehensive about the junior high experience. We ask that you please listen to Andy's parents. We did, and because of that, our families have been so richly blessed. Please reconsider Andy's situation. All of us will feel much more confident if he is with some of his friends. Thank you.

Evidently Andy's young friends had heard the saying, "If there's no wind, row." They, too, wrote to the junior high principal on August 23, 1997:

We're writing about Andy. He has been given a schedule without any friends in his classes. At our school he was treated the same by everyone. At your school he won't have anyone to stick up for him. We know that the teachers he was given are the best ones for him. But teachers alone aren't going to make Andy a better student, he also needs friends to encourage him. He's also more comfortable with people he knows. It's also important to us that Andy does well. Some of us have known him for seven years. We don't want to see him have to be alone, not having any friends in his classes. (Sincerely, Dan, Nick, Paul, and Phil)

His family called junior high "The Middle Ages," where Andy was again placed in regular classes, where he continued to learn and to teach. By the second semester, the teachers had learned how to teach Andy and had also become cognizant of the fact that he could learn. At the close of seventh grade, Andy's mother wrote to his teachers, thanking them for "teaching him what he was able to learn, handling him firmly and well, and spending hours writing notes and devising plans, and trying out ideas." During that first junior high year Andy was introduced to the world of athletics, Shakespeare, Twain, Dickens, and the Greeks. He learned about cells and bacteria, responsibility, Native Americans, the solar system, shooting hoops, history, how to get into his locker, electricity, how to pay the bill at McDonalds, and the joy of junior high dances.

Andy's mother had already experienced the hormone-filled adolescent years first-hand with her older three children. Indeed, she continued to worry about peer support during his days at the junior high school where three elementary schools merged to form the larger junior high. "Her moment" came one day, though, during the finale of the Johnny Termain unit. The English/American studies integration culminated in a production in which the eighth graders *became* colonial people, complete with costumes, as they role modeled early American times. Andy and another boy walked into the gym late. Andy stood alone looking uncomfortable and out of place, as the other boy jumped up easily into the bleachers and disappeared in the crowd. "Several rows up and over, a group of boys I knew from the football team noticed Andy." His mother continued, "I saw the motion to come, and heard the 'ANDY!' all at once, and even faster, Andy jumped up to join them. Andy, the kid so afraid of climbing and heights, about flew up, and made it in time to catch the high fives that were awaiting him. There they sat, all in their colonial vests and white shirts, as loyal to one another as their colonial counterparts had been to their ideals and beliefs!"

YES! Her moment had come! She says, "Like the echoes of the clumping on the steps of the elementary school, the thoughts of his cabin mates at sixth grade camp, and the letter 'the guys' wrote at the beginning of seventh grade, this ordinary day in November will always remind me of what is right and good in the world, and of those teachers whose work made an extraordinary boy able to be an ordinary child in his school."

Winter can be wicked on any northern coast, as was Andy's eighth grade winter. He became very ill that February, finally having to be admitted to Pediatric Intensive Care Unit in Rainbow Babies and Children's Hospital in Cleveland (a half hour away). In the words of Andy's mother, "I was back to day one, when I had prayed to please just let me have him to take home. I was back to the health worries that I had thought were over and done. Back to being forced to concentrate on the scar on his chest as a not-so-silent reminder, back to watching oxygen levels, and breathing and heart rates on machines, and I didn't like it at all! When the guys heard where he was, they came. With hair slicked down and in their dress pants left over from game day, Dan, Nick, Paul, and Jagger visited. And they phoned Phil!"

One of Andy's most loyal friends, Phil, had just recently moved six hours away because of his dad's job transfer. So worried about Andy, he decided emails and calls were not sufficient; he asked his parents to make the trip back so that he could see Andy and let him know how much he cared. It is easy to see why Phil is so caring, with parents who loaded all five of his brothers and sisters into their van and drive six hours one way so Phil might see his sick friend! Andy's mother concludes, "When Andy was born I never thought he would have friends, let alone friends and allies like these! I don't know that he will always have the friendships, the camaraderie he has now. But, for now, I will celebrate quietly in my heart, the ordinariness of friendships as prescriptives . . . and of life itself!"

The Middle Ages were not total joy, as Andy's mother writes (on behalf of future Andys who perhaps may set their sails in new directions, even if they don't follow in his wake). "In the spring of his ninth grade when he was almost done with junior high, someone gave him an application for the National Junior Honor Society; he qualified based on his grades. I saw for the first time, all the opportunities he had missed. I realized that all those little things, that I had been content to ignore, really did add up. They all added up to the missed points necessary to qualify for the Honors Society. Looking back, Andy wanted to be in band as he was in sixth grade but it was a total disaster! **They could have said,** 'What can we do to make this work?' And when I asked about the school plays. The reply was, 'The kids like to have a polished production.' **They could have said,** 'Is there something that Andy would like to do to help with it?' When track season arrived in the spring he was so excited to finally be IN a sport, but he had to take in the note from the doctor saying 'no.' **They could have said,** 'Is there a way he could help out with the team in another way?' When he signed up for intramurals, he was assigned to an eighth grade team instead of with his own ninth graders. **They could have said,** 'We will change him to a ninth grade team, instead of saying they thought it wouldn't matter what grade he played with.' He loves to take pictures. **They could have said,** 'Could he take some for the yearbook?' He loves to clown around. **They could have said,** 'Come and be in the talent show.' He loves drawing. **They could have said,** 'Come, join the art club!'"

But no one did!

Chapter 5 - Riptide
High School Years

However, any joy that Andy did experience at junior high was swept away as fiercely as a northeaster when it was time to enter high school, the largest three-year high school in Ohio. After Andy's mother again finally convinced the school "powers" that Andy needed regular classes, one teacher never talked to him the entire first grading period, and another refused to have him in her class. It must have been the dark ages for these teachers who had not yet learned to respect diversity, had not yet learned that considerable research suggests that diversity and risk-taking, along with a sense of humor, is strongly associated with learning. Sadly, they had not yet learned that life and growth emerge from new and unusual ideas, that differences are not nuisances nor embarrassments, and that students are not wallpaper patterns.

At the end of his disastrous tenth grade, Andy's parents read from a script they had written for presentation at his 504 meeting. "To watch most of the teachers ignore his 504 plan and the information given them in a variety of forms has been, at the least, disappointing. They had meetings for which they were given substitutes (time off from their classes), they had letters and other communications from us, and they had instructions from 'higher ups' in the system. Yet, they ignored doing what they were quite clearly told to do. We realize that we can no longer stand back, be polite and nod understandingly at the difficulties the system is having, as we watch our son's plan be ignored. What is happening is not only frustrating and sad, but illegal.

"It is no longer going to be our problem what the union says, that makes some teachers think they do not have to follow a plan written for Andy, which is based on federal law (John Satoran from the Office of Civil Rights assured us that Federal Law takes precedence over local contractual agreements). It is no longer going to be our problem that therapists don't have time in their schedules to see him during his study hall. It is no longer going to be our problem that tutors do not know how to teach reading. It is no longer going to be our problem that there is no accountability for teachers who choose to ignore his plan either in the classroom or during extracurricular activities. We are putting the system on notice, that Andy's plan WILL be followed, in the classroom and in all school activities, and that his needs will be met. He has only two more years of school if he is to graduate with the kids he has been with all of these years, and we will not have those two precious years be wasted, as this one was. We need to have it clearly stated, to everyone who is involved in Andy's education, that his plan is not an option, that following it is as critical to the teachers, as it is to Andy. As parents and family, we are sorry that things happen that make following his plan difficult, and we do understand that life doesn't always go as you plan, but we are done listening to excuses. Enough is enough!"

An <u>anonymous</u> rebuttal, written by "the staff" at the high school, added to the furor of those northeastern gales. In part, they "requested the opportunity to evaluate Andy and to consider his need for special education and related services and to consider more intensively, the transition needs Andy has."

His parents, forever his chief advocates, turned the tide with their response. "As we read of your concerns about Andy, we were hurt that you did not communicate with us your concerns early on, so that we all could have worked together to make things better for him and for you. We disagree with your suggestions on having him evaluated and referred to special education. Our decision was made a *long* time ago, that we wanted Andy to have all the experiences all of our children have had; that includes going to school with their neighbors and friends. We look at special education as a service, not a place, and we believe that those services can be provided where the student is. We wonder what you would have had him miss? Biology? Then he would not have experienced Charles Darwin, DNA, insect collections, and leaf collections (his teacher used Andy's leaf collection as a model for others). College English? He would have missed <u>To Kill a Mockingbird,</u> <u>Of Mice and Men</u> and <u>Lord of the Flies</u>, the latter two <u>so</u> relevant to his life! And just for your information, statistics show that students who have been in special education programs have a very low employability rate. We believe that his future success will be enhanced because of his experiences in his general education classes. . .You never got to see the kind of learner Andy can be. But that is nothing that referring him to someone else will take care of. You might have tried hard to include him in your own way, but I urge you to look through his 504 plan, and see exactly what you did and did not do. If each teacher would follow that plan, you would share the vision we have for Andy. We are sorry you missed that experience!"

His parent advocates again felt they were treading in rough waters when they verbalized the fact that there was no room on the bus for Andy, a football trainer who had worked hard all season (even the 6 a.m. practices the last three weeks of summer vacation). He could only be a trainer because his heart was physically not strong enough to withstand the rigors of playing the game. His parents expressed that 98 players, 125 band members, 20 cheerleaders, 10 other trainers, a mascot, a junior mascot, 15 coaches, and 4 band directors (274 in total) all rode in the long caravan of buses from the league championship game; one did not -- the one with 47 chromosomes instead of 46. The trainer boy was quiet during the trip home with his parents. He only said, "I'd just rather be with my friends."

As a trainer for basketball he rode the bus with the team to the first round of tournament games. When the team went to another level, there was again no room on the bus for him. But he had the end-of-the-season awards night to which he looked forward. A snow day postponed it, and he was never told when it was rescheduled! The policy of the school district reads: "Educational programs and activities are provided without regard to race, color, national origin, sex, or disability."

At the end of Andy's first semester of his junior year, his parents continue writing to the superintendent, the high school principal, and grade level principal. With each new wave they are merely asking for the things that are listed in his 504 plan, both in his classes and in his activities. "For him, being a trainer, or being involved in Community Service are almost more important than what he learns in class," they conclude in several of their communiqués asking for accountability by the district.

However some at the high school were aware that learning seldom comes from sitting passively still in the water with the sails flapping! Moderate southern breezes again prevailed during the second semester of his junior year because of Susan, a God-sent speech therapist. In addition to teaching Andy how to handle many facets of high school life by himself, she went to his teachers and explained his language difficulties. As good therapists do, she asked what they were studying in class, and then incorporated the classroom language he would then need. She planned with teachers some specific things they could ask Andy in class and he rehearsed his possible answers with her, and she helped him with his presentations.

Andy's accomplishments with projects, papers, and presentations reflected this support from therapists, tutors, teachers, parents and his own hard work. One exemplar was his junior research paper and presentation entitled "Segregation's Last Stand: Kids with Disabilities." Who better than Andy could speak on the topic? His work begins:

> We learned in history that segregation doesn't work.
> Separating black people from white people caused a lot of trouble.
> Putting Japanese-Americans in camps in World War II was not a good idea.
> The United States Supreme Court said that separate schools are not equal schools.
> But kids with disabilities like mine are usually segregated into separate classes or schools.
> They miss out on a lot of things.
> But not me. I am lucky. I am in regular classes!

What is important about people - and about schools - is what is different, not what is the same (Barth 1996).

As Sinatra sang, "The summer wind came blowin' in from across the sea, it lingered there so warm and fair" during Andy's senior year. Andy's mother writes to the new superintendent at graduation time, "When we saw what a difference Susan made, we again tasted the importance of support for included students, if inclusion is to be done right. Susan continued to work successfully with Andy, as did his college English teacher and his photography teacher, among others. We had a surprise when she put one of Andy's pictures in the display case in the hall, not because it was Andy's, but because it was good!"

His senior college English presentations were remarkable. During his first semester he created a beautifully illustrated project, "Observations on Art and Literature," combining his skills as a photographer with his knowledge of English literature. In the spring he wrote about another subject dear to his heart, "The Making of Athletic Trainers." For his oral presentation, Andy began: "Doc Woods is my name. Baseball is my game. I was the Babe's trainer. Babe as in Babe Ruth." His working portfolio, "How Do I Know What I Think until I See What I Say," contains examples of his continuous writing improvement from seventh through twelfth grades.

Along with the widening ripple of successful academics, his circle of friends continued to expand. When he asked one of his fellow trainers to go to the Homecoming Dance, she said she would love to, and later she was voted Homecoming Queen! He was part of that wonderful football season when the school went to the State of Ohio playoffs (for this year the head trainer finally allowed him to ride the bus to away games)! At the final Football Banquet, he stood proud and tall on the Fine Arts Center stage with all the other players and trainers. He introduced his parents to the audience as he presented his Mother with a rose - just like all the other athletes!

"It has been our goal to have Andy be just one of the kids," Andy's mother relates. "He has worked so hard to be just that. When we think of the homework he has done every single night, the weekends spent on projects and papers, and the hours getting presentations ready, we are amazed that he stuck it out. We remember the years he was sick more than well, when he did school work in the hospital and at home even though he felt so sick, and the days he went to school just because he couldn't miss any more. He is one tough boy!"

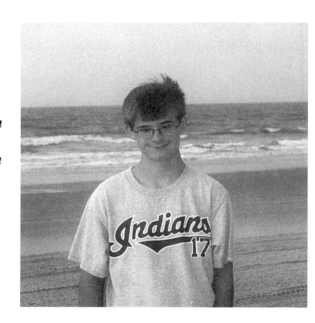

This part of his journey ended at the ceremony on June 7, 2003, when he donned his cap and gown for the graduation from Mentor High School.

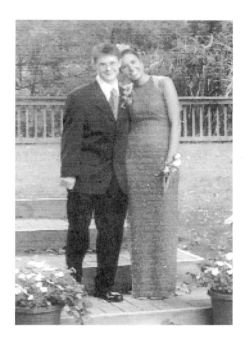

A night to remember!
Andy escorts Homecoming Queen Ashley
to the dance

Adorned in his honor cords
on Graduation Day!

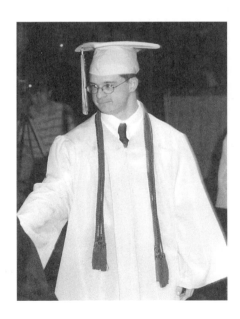

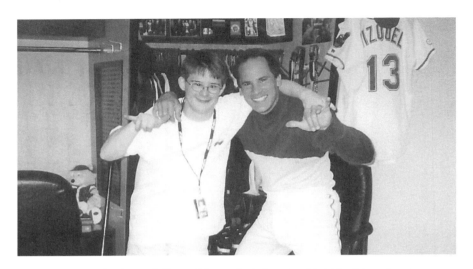

Andy and Omar Vizquel at Jacobs Field in Cleveland

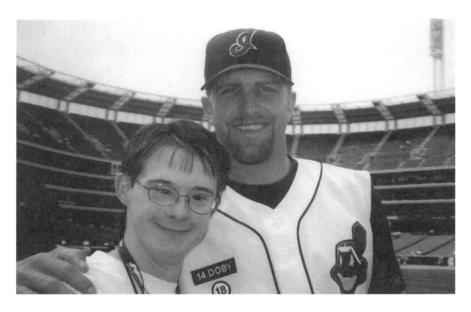

Andy and Casey Blake at the Jake

Chapter 6 - High Tide
Celebration

"And now it is the end. Except for Prom and Senior Project (with the Cleveland Indians trainers)," his mother continues. "A highlight was at Senior Honors Night when he received three honor cords; one for community service, one for his senior project, and one for graduating cum laude, all presented by the President of the Mentor Exempted Board of Education. They didn't understand my tears!"

Another highlight, this one for his elementary principal, was a graduation announcement from Andy, a cum laude student among 817 graduates in the Class of 2003. A humble note was tucked inside from mom who says, "He has really made us proud, hasn't he? And you were the one who opened the door for him. You didn't just let him come to Center Street Village School; you welcomed him. We will never forget all that you did for him."

Just as dependable as the tide, Andy will continue his journey, with favorable breezes at his back. He will continue within a circle of support which creates a community of reflection, growth, and refinement of practice. This circle of support sails smoothly with a rudder of strength, determination, and love, which continuously blossoms! For indeed, only those who risk going too far, exemplified by those in his dedicated circle of support, will ever know how far they can go.

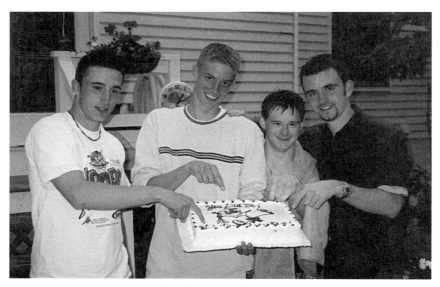

Graduates celebrate!
WJ, Nick, Andy and Phil

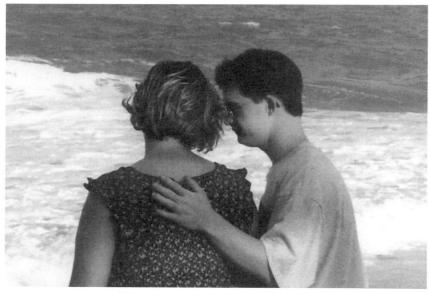

"The summer wind keeps blowin'
in from across the sea . . ."

Epilogue

Andy is now 21 years old and a student at Lakeland Community College in Kirtland, Ohio. In addition to his studies, he is manager of the men's basketball team. He is an avid Cleveland Indians fan, and hopes for a future job in a sports related field. Surrounded by a loyal group of friends, he is enjoying life in the real world as envisioned by his family and educators when the journey first began.

QUICK ORDER FORM

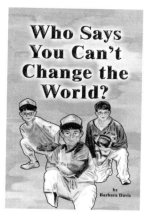

Barbara Davis offers her book as a living inspiration to all who have been touched by anyone with a disability. "Who Says You Can't Change the World?" shouts from the front of Andy's shirt. He wears it his first day of kindergarten in the neighborhood public school. His education journey is propelled through a sea of love and faith from his family, his teachers and other school personnel, his church and his community. Andy attended kindergarten through twelfth grade each day in regular classes despite his irregular chromosome count of 47 which results in Down syndrome. As he learned from his teachers along with his classmates each year, Andy subtly taught them how to be kinder and gentler humans. He taught them compassion and caring. Indeed, as long as you can change people, you can change the world!

Additional copies of *Who Says You Can't Change the World?* may be ordered using this form.

Hardcover $19.99
Paperback $11.99

Add $4.00 shipping for single copies and $2.00 for each additional book. Send check with order form below to:

BARBARA DAVIS
7293 BEECHWOOD DRIVE
MENTOR, OH 44060
PHONE: (440) 255-8015

Ambrosia Press
ambrosia03@earthlink.net

Name: _____
Address: _____
City: _____ State: _____ Zip: _____

_____ Qty. Hardcover @ $19.99   Total Hardcover $_____
_____ Qty. Paperback @ $11.99   Total Paperback $_____
                                     Shipping $_____

Who Says You Can't Change World?   **Total Enclosed** $_____

ACKNOWLEDGEMENTS

Many professionals, teachers, and staff in Mentor, Ohio, have worked hard to share in Andy's success story. "William Hiller, former Center Street Village School Principal and Mentor Schools Superintendent, presented possibilities to us regarding Andy's education. "Ron Patrick, director of psychological services, supported us all with his kind heart, generous spirit, and positive affirmation of our view of the future.

The teachers and staff who worked with him on a daily basis cannot go unnamed. They have done far more than what was required of them, not just for Andy, but for all the students who have had the good fortune to be in their classes. There was no manual to tell the people how to teach Andy. These individuals were willing to take things as they came and dealt with whatever each day brought. They were creative and understanding. They maintained their sense of humor as they taught him what he was to learn. They have made such a difference in Andy's life," comments Andy's mother. She continues her acknowledgements:

Mentor United Methodist Preschool:

Bonnie Newman
Paula Coleman
Janet Lewis
Linda Godek

Center Street Village School:

Sharon Kastor taught him to follow the rules;
Leslie Landis taught him to come in from the playground when it was time;
Jane Wink taught him reading, numbers, and success;
Bonnie Carlson taught him metamorphosis, and that letting go is part of life;
Linda Richards taught him to go with the flow;
Christine Harris taught him to write out his thoughts;
Laurie Kiss taught him his life was unique through writing his own autobiography;
Patricia Channel taught him that projects are a wonderful way to learn;
David Porter taught him about the pyramids, hieroglyphics, and Leonardo DaVinci;
Gloria Kilfoyle taught him to read, and to speak in front of the entire school;
Rose Dombos, who rewrote entire books for Andy, taught all of us to adapt curriculum;
Debbie Deal taught him to read music and play in the band as a percussionist;
Betty Krejsa taught him to appreciate great works of art; and,
Shirley Barker taught him telephoning by letting him call home often.

Ridge Junior High School:

Tim O'Keefe 8th/ 9th grade principal, welcomed all his students' challenges,
    providing for their success;
Stephen Heller welcomed him to the world of athletics;
John Williams taught him about cells, bacteria, and creatures that live in the sea;
Tracy Coleman introduced him to Mark Twain, Charles Dickens, and the Titanic;
Chris Parsons took him around the world and back, and taught him hat hard work
    brings rewards, like a Social Studies Department Award;
Laura Hoffman taught him to shoot hoops with "nothing but net";
Coach Lynch taught him responsibility, making him keeper of the keys to the locker room;
Connie Minerovic taught him words he needed to talk to his Spanish sister-in-law;
Jeff Perry taught him that hard work makes success no matter what the score;
Cindy Guest taught him to multiply and divide, and to pay the bill at McDonalds;
Sharon Curritt taught him how literature and history tell our story;
Lee Dreifort taught him that we have to learn from history, or it will repeat itself;
Kim Coolbaugh taught him about the stars, moon, planets, and the whole universe;
Wendy Luciano taught him about energy, electricity, and the Periodic Table; and,
Larry Luciano introduced him to Shakespeare, the Greeks, and research papers.

Mentor High School:

Susan Bleck taught him classroom language and so much more;
Ruth Erb was his tutor, advisor and friend;
Sharon Oleksak taught him how to take care of himself and those he loves;
Terry Molley taught him about his favorite novel, To Kill a Mockingbird;
Scott McLaughlin asked for a second chance so he could teach Andy better;
Carrie Banks cherished his presence in her classroom, and taught him about nutrition;
Donna Kohn allowed him to do his best by expecting nothing less;
Steve Trivisonno welcomed him into the football world, even as a lowly trainer;
Bob Krizancic allowed him to shoot around with the team, making him really belong;
Carol Cvar taught him how to do a job right by using him as an office aid for three years;
Kathy O'Connor helped him capture his precious moments on black and white film; and,
Terry Quigney always took care of the details that made Andy's high school life complete.

The author would like to share her deepest appreciation to some special people:
    To daughters Beth Ann Davis for her technical knowledge and patience
        and Polly D. Spaeth for her marketing management;
    To Nick Meyer for his talent and design in making Andy a visual
        reality through his cover art;
    To friends Gayle Shaw Cramer and Anne Morgan for their
        encouragement, inspiration and literary critiques;
    To Ambrosia Press Publisher Ruth Fawcett for patiently providing a
        path to follow; and
    To Paula Patterson for her inspiration, her creativity, her
        enrichment of the book through her writing, and for sharing
        her gift, Andy.

Watertown,__Wisconsin: Apple   Publishing   Company, Subsidiary   of Educational Assessment Service, Inc..

Rogers, Richard & Hammerstein, Oscar. (1949). You've got to be carefully taught, from the play, "South Pacific."
www.turnofftheviolence.org/Carefully taught.htm.

Webber,   Andrew   Lloyd.   (1986)   "Phantom   of   the   Opera," musicalization of the Gaston Leroux novel: London

Reprinted from <u>Phi Delta Kappan</u>, March 1990, ...

Bonde, Richard. (2003, June) Special education law. Unpublished journal by Lake Erie College, Painesville, OH. p.24.

Ibid. p. 26

Ibid. p. 31

Brooks, Garth. Standing outside the fire. Allspirit lywww.allspirit.co.uk/fire.html.

Bush, President George. Address presented to Federally Recognized Blue Ribbon Schools, September 17, 1990. The White House (South Lawn).

Dirck, Joe. (1991, May 2). Down pupils thriving in regular class. <u>The Cleveland Plain Dealer,</u> commentary.

Ellis, Frank K. (1968) <u>No man walks alone.</u> Westwood, New Jersey: Fleming H. Revell Company, 127.

Fulghum, Robert. <u>All I really need to know I learned in kindergarten.</u> New York: Ivy House.

Koff, Stephen. (2003, June 26). Pledge for disabled pupils cut in half. <u>The Cleveland Plain Dealer</u>, A-9.

Mathis, William J. (2003). No child left behind: Costs and benefits. <u>Phi Delta Kappan, 84</u>, 679-686.McClellan-Copeland, April. (1995, May 27). Students ponder Flanders Fields: Ceremony caps lesson on wars. <u>The Cleveland Plain Dealer,</u> 2-B.

I know Barbara Davis as an experienced educator and fluent author of articles in her field. The child-centered approach common to all her work is eloquently expressed in <u>Who Says You Can't Change the World?</u> An account of Barbara's involvement in the life of a special-needs student, it is a poignant case study of the exceptional collaboration between a family and the school to surround the child with every opportunity for success. Any parent or teacher can draw inspiration from this highly readable and engaging journey through Andy's developmental years.

Ruth Fawcett, Author/Publisher

* * * * *

Barbara Davis and I were both fortunate to be principals of America's Blue Ribbon elementary schools. When I read the application Barbara submitted for this award, I praised her for the way she had with words and her ability to tell a story. As an author, I truly appreciate a gifted writer. Now, after reading <u>Who Says You Can't Change the World?</u>, I put Barbara Davis in the category of gifted writer. I believe her book will help change the world by telling Andy's story.

Gayle Shaw Cramer, Author/Educator

* * * * *

It was great to receive your book, <u>Who Says You Can't Change the World?</u> Gary and I read it already because we really did not put it down once we started. Very inspiring, warm, emotional, and something everyone working with children should read and realize how powerful the way our kids are treated from the first moment makes such a difference. As we read through it, so many students, past and present, kept coming to mind. I will share our copy with our special education supervisor who will absolutely love it, as we did. She works constantly at making inclusion work well in our building and throughout the district.

The importance of Andy's story being told will continue to make a difference. Fantastic! Thanks for telling it for all the "Andys" in our schools.

Janet A. Larese, Assistant Principal
Westfield South Middle School, Westfield, MA

* * * * * *

Thank you, Mrs. Davis, for coming to Mentor Borders this Saturday. I'm so happy it went so well, and that Andy was able to come and autograph with you. You were a HUGE success. You touched many hearts. Thank you for being so kind and gracious.

Irene Sullivan, Bookseller

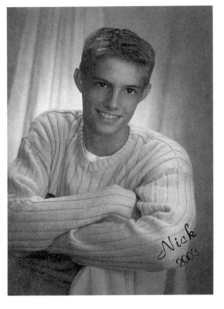

Cover design artist, **NICK MEYER**, is a junior art education major at Baldwin Wallace College (Berea, OH), as well as a first string basketball player. "Nick is a special well-rounded person with a good head on his shoulders. His 20-year friendship with Andy has played a paramount role in his enrichment and growth as a young adult," says Nick's mother. An excellent student, Nick learned loyalty and compassion, and through his special friendship with Andy he realized early on that people are more alike than different. "The children in that class have a special bond," according to Mrs. Meyer. "They learned to watch out for each other, they protected each other, even disciplined one another." When this author emailed Andy's mother for suggestions for a cover artist, her reply was, "YES! ONE WORD! NICK!"